# The Practical Guide to Extended Nurse Prescribing

*Christine Otway*

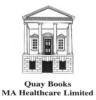

**Quay Books**
**MA Healthcare Limited**

Quay Books Division, MA Healthcare Limited, Jesses Farm, Snow Hill, Dinton,
Salisbury, Wiltshire, SP3 5HN

British Library Cataloguing-in-Publication Data
A catalogue record is available for this book

© MA Healthcare Limited 2004
ISBN 1 85642 232 1

Printed in the UK by Cromwell Press, Trowbridge

# Contents

# Contributors

Nicky Brooks M Phil, BSc (Hons) DPSN, RGN is a Research Co-ordinator in primary care at De Montfort University, Leicester. Her background is in intensive care nursing and practice development. In her last post as research fellow she undertook research into patients' perspectives of nurse prescribing. She has also researched the use of patient group directions in an NHS walk-in centre.

David Spence BSc (Hons), MRPharmS is a Public Health Specialist in Medicines Management with Eastern Leicester Primary Care Trust. He was previously pharmaceutical advisor to Leicestershire Health Authority. Despite being extremely busy he took time to contribute to this book.

## Acknowledgements

I would like to thank both contributors for their work.

Particular thanks to Nicky Brooks for her time and patience in reviewing and supporting me throughout and also to Jayne Morgan for reading and commenting on the book.

Also thanks to my husband, Kevin and daughter, Sally for their endless patience.

# Preface

If, on a regular basis, you find yourself going to the doctor you work with, and asking him to write a prescription for a patient who you have seen and assessed; or if you find yourself writing prescriptions for patients and waiting outside consulting room doors for your medical colleague to sign those prescriptions, then, after reading and considering the issues raised in this book, you should consider enrolling for the next nurse-prescribing course in your area. If you are unsure which course is the right one for you and your patients, read on!

If you are not a nurse and do not understand why nurses would want or need to prescribe, this book will answer your questions. The needs of the patient are at the heart of the nurse prescribing initiative and have been a core consideration in the planning and development of nurse prescribing from its inception. Patient needs have been a central consideration in the way this book has been constructed and is considered in every chapter.

(Nurses, midwives and health visitors will be referred to as nurses for the rest of this book. The female gender will also be used with apologies to male nurses, midwives and health visitors. This way of referring to nurses in general is for ease of writing and is not intended to cause offence to my respected colleagues of all disciplines and genders)

Christine Otway
September, 2003

# Introduction

This book is intended as a guide for those nurses, midwives or health visitors who are about to embark upon a nurse-prescribing course or for those involved in supplying or administering medications under patient group directions. It is also a useful guide for those who work with nurse prescribers and those who want to know more about this important initiative.

The book is chiefly concerned, as the title indicates, with the practicalities of prescribing, but in order to do this it looks firstly at the theoretical perspectives. The text commences with an historical overview of the development of nurse prescribing, considering why nurses might need to extend their practice to include prescribing skills. It also considers prescribing from the perspective of the patient.

*Chapter 2* considers the different ways that patients might access medications, setting nurse prescribing in the wider context. It looks at the part the nurse plays in extending the patients access to medications, detailing:

⌘ District nurse and health visitor nurse prescribing (DN and HVPX)
⌘ Independent extended nurse prescribing (IENPX)
⌘ Supplementary prescribing (SPX).

It also looks at the supply and administration of medicines under:

⌘ Patient group directions (PGDs).

The advantages and disadvantages of repeat prescribing are examined and other ways in which the general public access medications are highlighted.

Having decided that the nurse does need to become a prescriber, *Chapter 3* looks at what qualifications the nurse needs, and which courses are the most relevant to access in preparation for prescribing for their patients' needs. It also examines content of courses and time needed to study and prepare for practice. This is related to the support of management needed to embark on study and will help nurses and managers decide whether the amount of time needed to prepare to prescribe is warranted when weighed up against the likely benefits afforded to patients.

*Chapter 4* questions how nurses will maintain satisfactory levels of competence in the future and who and what will support them in this task. The place of clinical supervision, peer support, appraisals and personal development plans are examined. Information sources such as information technology (IT), journals and newsletters, the roles of the National Prescribing Centre (NPC) and the Prescription Pricing Authority (PPA) are also reviewed.

*Chapter 5* examines the ethical, accountability and legal issues which surround prescribing practice and suggests how these issues can be considered during each and every prescribing decision the nurse makes.

*Chapter 6* is a practical section, which gives a step-by-step guide to prescription writing. This section includes explanations for why codes must be correctly written and helps the nurse to avoid some of the common pitfalls in prescription errors.

*Chapter 7* looks at the particular issues involved in prescribing in a team context, looking at the various roles and responsibilities of:

- the independent prescriber
- the supplementary prescriber
- the patient
- non-prescribing nurse colleagues
- the nurse prescribing lead nurse
- the pharmacy advisor
- the community and hospital pharmacist
- the pharmacy technician
- the general practitioner (GP).

The book concludes in *Chapter 8* with a review of current developments and looks at the ways prescribing might be developed in the future.

Christine Otway
September 2003

# 1

# Why do nurses need to prescribe?

Many nurses have asked this question and answered it with one of the following responses:

> *We don't need to take on anything else.*
> *We don't have time.*
> *We are not doctors — we are nurses and why should we prescribe anyway.*

Fortunately, many nurses have taken a more positive stance and have realised that the ability to prescribe adds rather than detracts from the core unique function of the nurse. This function was one defined by Henderson (1991):

> *To assist the individual, sick or well, in the performance of those activities contributing to health or its recovery (or to a peaceful death) that he would perform unaided if he had the necessary strength, will or knowledge and to do this in such a way as to help him gain independence as soon as possible.*

Prescribing is an intrinsic part of this function and prescribable items and medicines are part of the essential items a nurse needs to carry this out. If a nurse knows exactly what a patient needs either to aid recovery or die with dignity, and if the ability to prescribe will enable her to carry out her nursing role, it follows that prescribing is a nursing task: not one which should remain in the exclusive domain of the doctor.

The general public are often unaware that nurses are not actually prescribers because their traditional role clearly involves the use of medications, enemas and dressings, which the public would not expect the nurse to have to obtain via a doctor (Fellows, 1999). Generally, patients are unaware of this situation until they are inconvenienced by the need to visit the doctor when the nurse has identified a need for a prescription (Anderson, 1999). Evidence of this perception by some patients has been identified by research into patients' perceptions of nurse prescribing (Brooks *et al*, 2001).

Nurse prescribing is about nurses taking responsibility for their own decision-making, improving their skills and increasing their knowledge base in order to prescribe effectively. It is also about nurses being fully aware of the legal and ethical issues which influence their choices and then accepting accountability for their own practice. In reality, it is very much about those issues which nurses consider in their core practice every day of their working lives. Nurse prescribing has enabled the expansion of nursing practice in areas where nurses have taken the lead: intermediate care, walk-in centres and nurse-led speciality areas, such as dermatology and respiratory care.

Not every nurse needs or wishes to prescribe independently, but there are many nurses who have clearly not yet considered their position on the subject. Until very recently, the options available for nurse prescribing did not apply to the majority of nurses because the extended formulary is limited to four major areas:

- minor ailments
- minor injuries
- health promotion
- palliative care.

It is, therefore, useful to nurses who specialise in any of these four areas. With the advent of supplementary prescribing (Department of Health [DoH], 2002) there is now an excellent opportunity for many more nurses to become prescribers. Supplementary prescribing is useful for specialist nurses, particularly those who work in areas of chronic disease management.

## Historical overview

Traditionally, it had always been doctors who prescribed, pharmacists who dispensed and nurses who administered medication (DoH, 1999). These traditional roles gradually became more blurred towards the end of the twentieth century, particularly in primary care, as nurses expanded their roles into nurse-led initiatives, such as NHS Direct, Hospital at Home, walk-in centres and intermediate care schemes. It could be argued that nurses, to a greater or lesser extent, had always been involved in the prescribing process, but as they became more aware of their own accountability and challenged by stepping outside of their traditional roles, it became clear that a legislative change was needed to keep pace with the extension of practice, in order to improve and develop nursing practice.

Nurses initially raised the issue of prescribing in 1978 through their professional forum, the Royal College of Nursing (RCN), in a report 'Nurses Dressings'. In 1985, a review of community nursing was conducted by a team led by Julia Cumberlege. The report which followed this review was formally titled *Neighbourhood Nursing: A focus for care*, but was informally known as the Cumberlege report (Department of Health and Social Security [DHSS], 1986). Publication of this report opened the debate on several innovative developments for nurses, many of which have been implemented (Cumberlege, 2003). Nurse prescribing was probably one of the most controversial of these developments at the time and although there was a great deal of support, there was also opposition from both within and outside the nursing profession. Doctors, who had been happy to countersign scripts written by nurses, were wary of letting go of their perceived control of the prescribing process. The British Medical Association (BMA) was opposed to any change and did not believe that nurse prescribing would ever be considered seriously (Cumberlege, 2003), with many nurses being reluctant to take a step further into a new area of responsibility. In order to improve access to medicines for patients it was becoming obvious that changes had to be made to the prescribing system.

The Government commissioned another team, this time led by Dr June Crown, to review the findings of the Cumberlege report and in 1989 the Crown report (DoH, 1989) recommended that nurses should be permitted to prescribe from a limited list of medicines, dressings and appliances. This report also recommended that nurses, doctors and pharmacists should collaborate in drawing up protocols, later to be known as patient group directions (PGDs), to facilitate easy supply of medicines to groups of patients with similar needs in defined situations (*Chapter 2*).

The anticipated benefits from nurse prescribing would be:

- improved use of both patient's and nurses time
- improved quality of care
- improved team working between health professionals.

The most significant concerns raised over implementing nurse prescribing were cost implications and an accountancy firm, Touche Ross, was requested to undertake a cost analysis (DoH, 1991). Further benefits were identified through this study, ie. that the savings made in terms of time and convenience for both health professionals and patients would offset costs of training nurses. The additional advantage identified would be a more rapid access for patients and increased job satisfaction for nurses. In March 1992, the primary legislation 'Medicinal Products: Prescription by Nurses'

Act was passed, but it was not until October 1994 that the necessary secondary legislation, the Medicinal Prescription by Nurses etc (Commencement No 1) Order 1994 came into effect.

In September 1994, the first fifty-eight nurses were trained to prescribe. These first nurses had to hold either the HV or DN qualification and be working as either practice nurses, health visitors or district nurses. It had taken fourteen years to arrive at this point and it was not until 1999, over twenty years after the debate started, that nurse prescribing was finally rolled out. Every qualified health visitor (HV), district nurse (DN) or practice nurse (PN) who held either of these community qualifications, was trained to prescribe as part of their specialist training course. This difficult progress has been described as one of the 'hardest fought battles of nursing' (Jones, 1999).

Evaluations of early nurse prescribing were generally positive (Luker, 1997). Following an extensive consultation exercise the second Crown report (DoH, 1999b) recommended a further expansion of nurse prescribing to other groups of first level registered nurses. It also recommended an expansion of the formulary. In August 2000, a health service circular detailed how nurses and pharmacists could legally supply and administer medicines under patient group directions (PGDs). These plans had previously been known as group protocols. Patient group directions permit the supply of particular medicines to specific groups of patients, who present for care without having previously been identified for treatment (DoH, 2000a). A nurse or another health professional, such as a paramedic or a pharmacist, might provide care in this instance. The medicine, the type of patient, the type of health professional and the qualifications they must hold, should all be specified with the patient group direction.

In May 2001, an announcement was made that nurses who had completed a recognised training programme at an institute of higher education would be permitted to prescribe all licensed 'general sales list' medicines and appliances (GSLs), all licensed 'pharmacy' medicines and one hundred and forty prescription only medications (POMs) from an 'Extended Nurse Prescribers Formulary'.

The English National Board for Nursing, Midwifery and Health Visiting (ENB) were asked to determine the standard, kind and content of educational preparation that nurses would require to prepare them to prescribe from the *Extended Nurse Prescribers' Formulary*. Higher education institutes (HEIs) then designed courses, which had to meet the criteria and be successfully validated by the ENB in order to prepare nurses for professional registration as extended independent nurse prescribers. Initially, it was decided that these courses must include twenty-five taught days in university and twelve days of medical supervision in practice, to be delivered within three months. In order to meet the *NHS Plan* (DoH, 2000b) targets, the Government were keen for these courses to start as soon as possible, as were prospective students keen to commence training. In some parts of England courses started in January or February 2002. Initial experience of these courses indicated that the timescale was very tight and the ability to meet learning outcomes in practice was difficult. In October 2002, in response to difficulties articulated by HEIs and service managers, the Nursing and Midwifery Council (NMC) changed the directive set by the English National Board (ENB) that the course must be run over three months. Universities had the opportunity to extend the courses over any period between three and six months. This change was to enable more nurses to be released from practice to attend courses, as well as meeting their obligations to meet service requirements.

At the same time as extended nurse prescribing was being implemented another consultation exercise was taking place. Between April and July 2002, proposals to develop supplementary prescribing for nurses and other health professionals were considered (DoH, 2002). This consultation was a direct result of the recommendations made in the Crown 2 report (DoH, 1999b) and even earlier recommendations made in the Cumberlege report (DHSS, 1986) that nurses should be able to alter dosages and timings of medications within an agreed treatment plan as dependent prescribers. The term 'supplementary' prescribing superseded the term 'dependent' prescribing and NHS organisations, as well as individuals, were asked for their comments on the Department of Health proposals.

The legal premise for introducing supplementary prescribing had been facilitated by the Health and Social Care Act 2001 Section 63, which allows ministers by order to designate new categories of prescriber and to set conditions for their prescribing. Amendments to the 'prescription only medicines' order and changes to NHS regulations allow nurses and pharmacists who have been appropriately trained to prescribe

On 21 November, 2002 an announcement by Lord Hunt declared that nurses and pharmacists would be the first group of professionals to be able to train as supplementary prescribers. By this time, the ENB and United Kingdom Central Council for Nurses, Midwives and Health Visitors (UKCC) had been replaced by the Nursing and Midwifery Council (NMC) and the NMC were therefore charged with the task of advising on the standard of preparation, which would be required for supplementary prescribing. The NMC created standards for the preparation of nurses, midwives and health visitors (*Appendix II*) and the British Pharmaceutical Society were asked to take on similar task for pharmacists. The Department of Health created guidance for practitioners (www.doh.gov.uk/supplementaryprescribing/index.htm prescribing) and an implementation guide was written (DoH, 2003) and circulated to all NHS organisations.

It was decided that the newly developed EINPX courses fulfilled most of the requirements for the knowledge base needed for nurses to become supplementary prescribers with the addition of a further module. This meant that existing EINPX courses could be extended by one to two days and supplementary prescribing could be integrated successfully. Existing extended independent nurse prescribers, of which there were at the time between 500 and 800, were able to return to university for one to two days to 'top up' their existing qualification to become supplementary prescribers.

Nurses who trained as extended independent and later supplementary prescribers were identified by an annotation to their NMC registration indicating that they were extended nurse prescribers.

## The patient's perspective

### The policy context

In order to meet the needs of patients, boundaries of clinical work are being redrawn, most notably between doctors and nurses. A complex mixture of pressures coming from new technologies, treatments, changing patterns of health and social care and the processes by which services are purchased and provided has contributed to this. This has been supported by current policy; interprofessional working being highlighted as a means of modernising the NHS. *Working Together − Securing a quality workforce for the NHS* (DOH, 2000c) charges local healthcare providers with the tasks of recruiting and retaining a workforce with 'capacity, skills, diversity and flexibility' to meet the needs of the NHS in the twenty-first century.

Nurse prescribing is at the conjunction of modernisation policies. *Making a Difference* (DoH, 1999) proposed the extension of nurse prescribing, which was also identified by the Chief Nursing Officer as one of the key roles for nurses. The driving force behind these changes clearly is to meet patient need (Mullally, 2003):

> *To improve patients experience by providing fast, fair, convenient high quality services which respond to their needs.*

## The evidence to date

There were eight fund-holding practices recruited in 1994 for the nurse prescribing demonstration sites, one from each of the old regional health authorities. Four were from northern health authorities and four from the south. There was also a mixture of rural, urban and inner city practices, of which two were dispensing practices. Luker *et al* (1997) undertook the evaluation, which included a patient's/carer's perspective specifically around:

₭   Pre-prescribing — describe the methods by which patients/carers procure prescriptions, utilised in nursing care and the associated costs.
₭   Post-prescribing — to identify (social, emotional or financial) to the patients/carer as a results of nurse prescribing.

One hundred and fifty-seven patients were recruited pre-nurse prescribing, 148 patients were recruited post-prescribing of which fifty-seven participated in pre- and post-implementation interviews and were able to comment specifically on the changes. Patients were overwhelmingly in favour of the nurses' prescribing ability. The majority of patients were not aware of the nurses' new prescribing role, as the way in which they obtained their prescriptions did not change, ie. nurses often obtained items on patients' behalf or they received pharmacy deliveries. It was identified that general practitioners (GPs), nurses, patients and carers alike saved time. This was typified through reducing carers' journeys to collect the prescription and items and reduced patient time in having to book an appointment to see the GP and gaining quicker access to the prescribed treatment. Healthcare professionals' skills were used more appropriately as less time was spent having to wait for doctors to sign prescriptions.

Patients identified satisfaction around the nurse prescribing consultation process: nurse prescribers were seen as approachable, used the same language, and made the patients feel more relaxed. This may have been explained by the fact that the majority of the consultations took place in the patient's own home and the nurses were perceived to be more aware of the patient's individual circumstances. Nurse prescribing was linked to the individual nurse's personal qualities and skills, with patients identifying that not every nurse should be prescribing, ie. junior nurses. Conversely, there were areas in which the nurse was considered to be the more appropriate prescriber, for example, health visitors were seen to be the experts with young children.

There were few disadvantages identified apart from initial confusion over who could prescribe what, and if patients had a nurse and doctor prescribe the onus of the medical prescription was transferred to the patient. Patients reported that they quickly became familiar with this new method of working and became clear about the professional boundaries between the nurse and doctor.

Luker *et al's* (1997) evaluation was undertaken in the initial stages of the role out of independent nurse prescribing. Patients were reflecting upon 'novice prescribers.' The benefits may be underestimated as nurses grappled with the new world of prescribing. The richness of the data may have been affected by the methods used to capture patients perception's, ie. diaries. Alderman (1996), a community nurse involved in the demonstration project, identified that completing these diaries created problems for some of the older patients. There was little published information concerning the patients who participated in the evaluation. Although there was a mixture of urban and rural practices we do not know about the ethnic mix or socio-economic status of these patients, which may impact upon nurse prescribing. Finally, the patients were chosen as they were high users of community nursing services. The benefits of nurse prescribing may have been influenced by the continuing relationship between the nurse and the patient. It could be argued that prescribing practice is best within this type of relationship, ie. patient/GP.

**Brooks *et al*, 2001**

This study was undertaken in one primary care group in Leicestershire where the local trust had commenced its nurse prescribing training programme more than three years previously. Unlike Luker *et al* (1997), the nurse prescribers in this study which the patients reflected upon were more experienced. The aims of the study were to explore patients' reactions to/experiences of nurse prescribing, including acceptability, benefits and limitations/inconveniences. Fifty-four patients were recruited of which fifty participated in a semi-structured interview. The majority of patients were classified as new or low users of nurse prescribing in contrast to Luker's work, ie. they had received between one to three prescriptions.

The gains/benefits identified by patients included the following. Timeliness, 72% of the patients got an assessment and/or the prescription at the same time. This meant that the treatment could commence at once. Nurse prescribing was limited to minor treatments, so whether all participants treatment needed to start straight away and whether some ailments may have improved without a prescription is questionable. Timeliness of treatment does demonstrate evidence of flexible ways of working to provide better services for patients. The effective use of nurses' and doctors' time was the second most common theme identified by the patients (46 %). They recognised that minor problems were best dealt with by the nurse, enabling the GP to concentrate on more serious matters. Only two patients talked about nurse prescribing in terms of saving time for the nurse. Patients viewed nurse prescribing as more convenient (46%) as the care was centred on patients' needs, usually in their own homes. The relationship they had with the nurse prescriber was viewed as a quality: the nurse was approachable, spoke the same language, provided reassurance and continuity. This may have impacted upon under-reporting patients feeling able to talk about what they perceive as relatively minor problems. The nurse was also perceived as expert within the realms of wound care, catheter care, nappy rash, mastitis, thrush, dry skin and eczema and other common complaints in mothers and babies. Patients were confident that nurses were aware of their professional limitations, for example, the nurse would be aware of when things should be referred to the GP and take the appropriate action. The nurse prescriber was also viewed as practical; being able to work with patients to solve, anticipate problems and know the quantities of products to supply and methods of delivery. The majority of patients had been unaware, like Luker *et al* (1997), that nurses could prescribe, which may have been symptomatic of assimilation into practice or a means of protecting workload, ie. if the patient doesn't know I can perform this role then they won't ask or expect it.

In terms of future improvements and/or limitations, 98% of the patients were happy with the process: the consultation and the effect of the prescription in remedying the problem. Patients reflected finally upon the limitations of nurse prescribing. Sixty-six percent were happy with nurse prescribing and unable to identify limitations. The remaining 34% were more experienced users of nurse prescribing and were perhaps more informed and critical. Terms and conditions were linked to any changes with future nurse prescribing. Patients talked about competence and training (again identified by Luker *et al*, 1997), differences between medical and nursing education and the need for nurses to undertake further training if prescribing was extended. Very few patients said nurses should be able to prescribe the same as doctors.

Some of the patients who identified limitations had other nurses providing care or could identify a role for nurse and pharmacists in prescribing. Continuity was a key word on patients' lips, with future areas for expansion, including repeat prescribing and prescribing from a wider formulary especially for the under fives.

This study was undertaken in a largely white locality with lower than average unemployment figures as compared to the county. The impact of nurse prescribing upon ethnicity and deprivation from the patient's perspective still remains fairly elusive. In terms of the economic issues alone, one might expect that nurse prescribing would be more beneficial to families who were economically disadvantaged, particularly as the *Nurse Prescribers' Formulary* contained a considerable amount of over the counter (OTC) items, such as paracetamol suspension. Twenty-seven nurse prescribers were asked to recruit five patients, for whom they had recently prescribed. This would have resulted in a sample size of 135 patients. Only fifty-four patients were recruited, which may have been a reflection of low prescribing activity or that nurses interpreted this as writing prescriptions rather than prescribing in its widest sense.

What is clear from these two pieces of published work around the patient's perspective of independent nurse prescribing, is the way in which patients have experienced and accepted this new role. Patients are becoming 'monitors' of new ways of healthcare delivery and will be increasingly influential in the way that nurses and other healthcare professionals work. The patient's perspective of independent nurse prescribing has been to date fairly limited, when you consider the nurse prescribing literature around healthcare professionals' perspectives and educational issues. This is surely set to change (in light of the recent policy emphasis, eg. DoH, 2001). With extended independent nurse prescribing roles, the patient at long last should be able to take centre stage and inform the future prescribing agenda.

# References

Alderman C (1996) Prescribing pioneers. *Nurs Standard* **10**(18): 26–7

Anderson P (1999) Looking at the road ahead for nurse prescribers. *Community Nurse* **5**(11): 35–6

Brooks N, Otway C, Rashid C, Kilty L, Maggs C (2001) Nurse prescribing — what do the patients think? *Nurs Standard* **15**(17): 33–8

Cumberlege J (2003) A triumph of sense over tradition: the development of nurse prescribing. *Nurse Prescribing* **1**(1)

Department of Health (2000) *The NHS Plan, A plan for investment, A plan for reform.* The Stationery Office, London

Department of Health and Social Security (1986) *Neighbourhood Nursing: A focus for care* (Cumberlege Report). The Sationery Office, London

Department of Health (1991) *Nurse Prescribing: A Final Report: A cost benefit study* (Touche Ross Report).(unpublished) DoH, London

Department of Health (1989) *Report on the Advisory Group on Nurse Prescribing* (Crown Report). The Stationery Office, London

Department of Health (1999a) *Making a difference. Strengthening the nursing, midwifery and health visiting contribution to health and healthcare.* The Stationery Office, London

Department of Health (1999b) Review of Prescribing, Supply and Administration Final Report (Crown 2). HMSO, London

Department of Health (2000a) Health Service Circular (2000/026): NHS Executive. *Patient Group Directions*. DoH, London

Department of Health (2000b) *The NHS Plan*. DoH, London

Department of Health (2000c) *Working Together — Securing a quality workforce for the NHS*. The Stationery Office, London

Department of Health (2001) *Involving Patients and the Public in Healthcare: discussion document*. DoH, London

Department of Health (2002) *Agenda for Change. A modernised NHS pay system*. The Stationery Office, London

Department of Health (2003) *Supplementary prescribing by nurses midwives and health visitors: An implementation guide*. The Stationery Office, London

Fellows P (1999) Nurse prescribing: Politics to practice. In: Jones M *The Medical Opinion*. Ballière Tindall, London: chap 2

Henderson V (1991) *The Nature of Nursing: Reflections after 25 years, a definition and its implications for practice, research and education*. National League for Nursing Press, New York

Jones M (1999) *Nurse Prescribing: Politics to Practice*. Ballière Tindall, London

Luker K, Austin L, Hogg C, Willock J, Wright K, Ferguson B *et al* (1997) *Evaluation of Nurse Prescribing Final Report*. Unpublished report. The University of Liverpool and The University of York

Mullally S (2003) *Keynote speech*. 5th Annual Association of Nurse Prescribers Conference 2003, Centennial Centre, Birmingham

## 2

# What are the options?

Prescribing medicines, dressings and appliances form the largest and most costly of all healthcare interventions (NPC, 2002), but until 1992 these interventions had to be authorised by a doctor. This inevitably involved delay for the patient and time wasting for nurses. The implementation of nurse prescribing for district nurses and health visitors had an impact on this situation and promoted the cause to extend both the formulary and the types of nurses able to use prescribing powers. This chapter examines the various other ways in which patients can access medicines and appliances.

## Classifications of medicines

The 1968 Medicines Act listed medicines into three categories:

- general sales list medicines (GSL)
- pharmacy medicines (P)
- prescription only medicines (POM)

General sales list medicines can be bought 'over the counter' (OTC) by members of the general public from a sales assistant in a pharmacy, shop, garage or a supermarket. An independent medical or extended independent nurse prescriber may prescribe licensed general sales list medicines. Some general sales list items are included in the district nurse (DN), health visitor (HV) prescribers' formulary, and supplementary prescribers (nurses or pharmacists) can also prescribe them if they are included in an individual clinical management plan for a specific patient.

A member of the general public can buy pharmacy (P) medicines over the counter, but they can only be bought under the supervision of a pharmacist. An independent medical or extended independent nurse prescriber may prescribe licensed pharmacy only medicines. Some of these items are included in the DN, HV prescribers' formulary (*NPF*) and supplementary prescribers (nurses or pharmacists) can also prescribe them if they are included in an individual clinical management plan for a specific patient.

Prescription only medicines (POMs), as the name suggests, can only be obtained on prescription from an independent or supplementary prescriber.

## Types of prescribers

### Definition

> *Independent prescribing means that the prescriber takes responsibility for the clinical assessment of the patient, establishing a diagnosis and the clinical management required, as well as for prescribing where necessary and the appropriateness of any prescription.*
>
> (DoH, 2003)

Prescribers fall into the following categories:

### *Independent medical prescribers*

Doctors, dentists and vetinary surgeons were the only professionals legally allowed to prescribe under the Medicines Act of 1968 until the legislation was changed in 1992 to include nurses. Independent medical prescribers prescribe from the *British National Formulary* (*BNF*) on an FP10 form, commonly known as a prescription pad in primary care settings and on a hospital drug chart or ward order in secondary care settings (more detail about prescribing can be found in *Chapter 6*).

### *Independent health visitor or district nurse prescribers*

Since the Prescription by Nurses Act 1992, health visitors and district nurses or practice nurses (PN) who have trained as district nurses or health visitors and completed the nurse prescribing course, or who trained as health visitors or district nurses after 1999, and have their prescribing qualification annotated on the NMC register, can prescribe from the limited *Nurse Prescribers Formulary* (*NPF*). This consists of appliances, dressings and some medicines, including twelve prescription only medicines (POMs). These nurses prescribe on an HV/DN prescription form, FP10P.

### *Independent extended nurse prescribers*

Since 2002, all first level nurses who have completed the recognised extended independent nurse prescribing training and have had their

Nursing and Midwifery Council registration annotated accordingly, can prescribe from the *Extended Nurse Prescribers' Formulary* (*BNF* 45). These nurses prescribe on an FP10P form, commonly known as an extended nurse prescriber prescription and on a hospital drug chart or ward order in secondary care settings. Hospital prescribers may also prescribe on internal hospital prescription forms where the prescription is to be dispensed by the hospital pharmacist for outpatients or on an FP10HP for outpatients where a community pharmacist will dispense the prescription. This may only be done when a local policy has been developed and where a stamp is available to endorse the prescription with the nurse prescribers' details and NMC number.

## Supplementary nurse prescribers

First level nurses who have completed the recognised extended independent and supplementary nurse prescribing training and have had their Nursing and Midwifery Council registration annotated accordingly, can prescribe any item from the *BNF*, currently excluding controlled drugs, or unlicensed medications which have been written in to an agreed clinical management plan (CMP) (DoH, 2003). The CMP has to be drawn up and signed in agreement with a doctor, who is the independent prescriber, the patient and the supplementary prescriber. The definition of supplementary prescribing is:

> *A voluntary prescribing partnership between an independent prescriber and a supplementary prescriber to implement an agreed patient specific clinical management plan with the patient's agreement.*

> (DoH, 2003)

## Supplementary pharmacist prescribers

Pharmacists who have completed the recognised pharmacist prescribing course and have had their registration annotated accordingly, will be able to prescribe any item from the *BNF*, excluding controlled drugs, as long as the drug has been included in an agreed clinical management plan (DoH, 2003). The CMP has to have been drawn up and signed in agreement between a doctor, who is the independent prescriber, the patient and the supplementary prescriber.

## Supply and administration under patient group directions

The Medicines Act of 1968 permits doctors, dentists and vets to prescribe prescription only medicines. This act also authorises other professional groups to administer prescription only medicines in accordance with the written or verbal direction of the medical practitioner. In accordance with this act, nurses have supplied and administered medication under 'group protocols' in areas including emergency hormonal contraception and immunisations (Britten, 1995).

Although group protocols had been used in practice for some time, their application had been interpreted in an ambiguous manner so that they included clinical guidelines and procedures as well as orders for the administration of medicines (Baird and Morgan, 2001). This practice was repeatedly brought into question culminating with the Crown Review (DoH, 1999), which developed stringent criteria and called for clarification of the law. This review made it clear that any changes to the way in which drugs were supplied or administered should still be, wherever possible, prescribed on an individually named patient basis; patient's safety should not in any way be compromised and the provision of medicines to patients should optimise professional expertise and effective use of resources.

In 2000, the Medicines Control Agency (MCA, 2000) released a consultation document as a lead up to the expected legal changes. For the first time the use of the term patient group directions (PGDs) was used. Patient group directions were made legal under secondary legislation introduced on 9 August, 2000. A patient group direction is defined as:

> *A specific written instruction for the supply or administration of named medicines in an identified clinical situation. It is drawn up locally by doctors, pharmacists and other appropriate professionals and approved by the employer, advised by the relevant professionals advisory committees. It applies to groups of patients or other service users who may not be individually identified before presentation for treatment.*
>
> (DoH, 1999)

In order to clarify this legal position, a health circular (NHS, 2000) was produced. According to this circular, all PGDs should include the following particulars:

⌘ The name and date of the business to which the direction applies.

⌘ The date the direction comes into existence and expires.

⌘ A description of the medicines to which the direction applies.

⌘ Class of health professionals who may administer the medicine.

⌘ Signature of a doctor or dentist as appropriate and a pharmacist.

⌘ Signature by an appropriate health organisation.

⌘ Clinical condition or situation to which the direction applies.

⌘ A description of those patients excluded from treatment under the direction.

⌘ A description of those circumstances in which further advice should be sought from a doctor and arrangements for referral.

⌘ Details of appropriate dosage, maximum total dosage, quantity, pharmaceutical form and strength, route and frequency of admission, and minimum and maximum period over which the medicine should be administered.

⌘ Relevant warnings, including potential adverse reactions.

⌘ Details of necessary follow-up actions and circumstances.

⌘ A statement of the records to be kept for audit purposes.

This legislation applies to the NHS in England only and includes health professionals ranging from nurses to optometrists to ambulance paramedics. These groups of staff can supply and administer medicines only as named individuals whose names appear on the PGD. Names of those involved in drawing up the PGD must also be included in the PGD.

Controlled drugs are currently prevented from inclusion on PGDs through the Misuse of Drugs Act 1971. However, the Medicines Control Agency and the Home Office are currently discussing the possibility of amending the regulations to include substances under schedules 4 and 5 under PGDs. At the time of writing, a consultation exercise is in progress.

For further information regarding patient group directions see: www.groupprotocols.org.uk/

## Repeat prescribing

The repeat prescribing system is a universal method used by general practitioners (GPs) to ensure that patients can obtain prescribable items which have been previously prescribed for them. The time between prescription repeats is usually set at intervals in the future, stipulated by the prescriber. The prescriber also sets a date for review of the original prescription. This would apply to ongoing conditions where there is unlikely to be a change of dosage or medication required. The patient is given their original prescription with a form attached, listing the items which might be requested as repeat prescription items. When the patient needs more supplies he or she simply completes the prescription request and returns it to the surgery. Most practices operate a forty-eight-hour turnaround system so the patient returns after forty-eight hours to collect their completed and signed prescription, without needing to see the GP.

In order for this system to work safely and efficiently there needs to be a control system in place so that the originally prescribed medications are reviewed regularly. Review of medication ensures cost and clinical effectiveness and may have some beneficial impact on the current wastage figure which, according to the Medicines Partnership website (NPC, 2002), is currently estimated to be around £100 million per year. Unfortunately, many practices have inadequate control systems in place (Zermansky, 1996; McGavcock, 1999). Attitudes of GPs tend to affect whether or not control systems are in place and high spending practices tend to be the worst offenders (Watkins *et al*, 2003). When control systems are not in place, issues such as poor compliance with medication tends to go unnoticed; but when repeat prescribing is well managed there are significant improvements in both cost and clinical effectiveness (Bond *et al*, 2000).

## Self-medication

A number of minor ailments, such as the symptoms of the common cold and minor injuries such as sprains or insect bites are effectively dealt with by the patient without the need to contact a doctor or a nurse. The local pharmacist is also easily accessible for patients to seek advice when purchasing 'over the counter' medications. Many members of the public also take herbal or homeopathic remedies or food supplements to increase their perceived health or well being (Henry, 1995). As self-medication is common, it is important that the nurse considers this when prescribing for a patient and includes these items when conducting a medication review.

## References

Baird A, Morgan J (2001) Developing a patient group direction for use in primary care. *Primary Health Care* **11**(1): 21–4

Britten N (1995) Patient demands for prescriptions in primary care. *Br Med J* **310**: 1084–5

Bond C, Matheson C, Williams S, Williams P, Donnan P (2000) Attitudes and behaviour of general practitioners and their prescribing costs: a national cross sectional survey. *Br J Gen Pract* **50**(453): 271–5

Department of Health (1999) *Review of Prescribing, Supply and Administration Final*. DoH, London

Department of Health (1999) Review of Prescribing, Supply and Administration Final Report (Crown 2). HMSO, London

Department of Health (2003) *Supplementary Prescribing: An Implementation Guide*. The Stationery Office. London

Department of Health (2003) Online at: www.doh.gov.uk/nurseprescribing (Last accessed 24 January 2003)

Henry J (1995) *Over the counter drugs The British Medical Association Guide to Medicines and Drugs*. Dorling Kindersley, London, New York, Stuttgart

Medicines Control Agency (2000) *Consultation Document: Patient Group Directions*. DoH, London

Medicines Control Agency (2001) *Extended Prescribing of Prescription only medicines by independent nurse prescribers*. MLX 273. DOH, London.

McGavock H,Wilson-Davis, Conolly JP (1999) Repeat prescribing management — a cause for concern? *Br J Gen Practice* **49**(422): 343–7

National Prescribing Centre (2002) *Signposts for Prescribing nurses*. CD Rom

NHS Executive (2000) *Patient group directions* (England only) HSC 2000/026. NHSE, Leeds

Watkins C, Harvey I, Carthy P, Moore I, Robinson E, Brawn R (2003) Attitudes and behaviour of general practitioners and their prescribing costs: a national cross-sectional survey. *Qual Saf Health Care* **12**(1): 29–34

Zermansky AG (1996) Who controls repeats? *Br J Gen Practice* **46**(412): 643–7

# 3

# How do I prepare to prescribe?

There are now several ways in which a nurse can prescribe but all of the ways apply only to level one registered nurses who have undertaken a recognised additional training course. This chapter describes the types of prescribing and the training required for each method.

## Health visitor and district nurse training

The preparation for prescribing from the health visitor (HV) or district nurse (DN) prescribers' formulary (*BNF*) has been an integral part of health visitor's and district nurse's training courses since the national roll out of nurse prescribing in 1999. Prescribing skills are assessed using a written examination or an assignment during the course, and assessed in practice by the community practice teacher or mentor.

Health visitors and district nurses who trained before 1999 attended three days of training, following twenty hours of self-directed study working from an open learning pack produced by the English National Board (ENB), and were required to pass a written examination in order to prescribe from the *Nurse Prescribers' Formulary*. Most of these early nurse prescribing courses have ceased to run, to the disadvantage of a few health visitors and district nurses who may have been out of practice during the period 1997–2000. Although at the time of writing the focus for nurse prescribing development in higher education institutions (HEIs) and elsewhere appears to be on extended independent and supplementary prescribers, we must not neglect to mention the significant and important role of these 23,000 DN and HV prescribers in England.

## Extended independent and supplementary prescribing

Courses were developed in several HEIs in accordance with the outline curriculum provided by the English National Board (*Appendix I*) (now adopted by the Nursing and Midwifery Council) and the Nursing and Midwifery Council Standards (*Appendix II*) for extended independent and supplementary prescribing by nurses, midwives and health visitors.

The extended nurse-prescribing course is a stand-alone professional course, which attracts twenty level 3 academic credits. The validating body, the ENB, defined this award and universities found their guidance was non-negotiable. Anecdotally, most universities were unhappy because the amount of contact hours and the rigorous assessment regulations warranted a higher award. The ENB also stipulated that the course would be delivered over a three-month period (twenty-five days theory in total), and the equivalent of one day per week (twelve days practice in total) practice-based experience under the supervision of a medical mentor. Learning outcomes were devised in accordance with the NMC standards (*Box 3.1*).

---

**Box 3.1: Learning outcomes for extended independent nurse prescribing:**

1. Undertake assessment and consultation with patients and carers.
2. Prescribe safely, appropriately and cost effectively.
3. Understand the legislation relevant to the practice of nurse prescribing.
4. Understand and use sources of information, advice and decision support in prescribing practice.
5. Understand the influences on prescribing practice.
6. Apply knowledge of drug actions in prescribing practice.
7. Understand the roles and relationships of others involved in prescribing, supplying and administering medicines.
8. Practice within a framework of professional accountability and responsibility in relation to nurse prescribing.

---

When the course was extended to include supplementary prescribing the learning outcomes reflected this integration (*Box 3.2*).

## Learning and teaching strategies

The range and type of strategies used in the delivery of the extended independent prescribing courses were not stipulated by the ENB and therefore universities could design their own courses as long as the learning outcomes were met. This enabled course management teams to be flexible and, in some cases, redesign some elements of courses to meet the needs of a very diverse student group. In practical terms, strategies were dictated by factors such as the size of the group, the topic being addressed, the learning environment and the available resources.

**Box 3.2: Learning outcomes for extended independent and supplementary nurse prescribing:**

1.  Undertake assessment and consultation with patients and carers.
2.  Analyse the suitability of patients' situations for either independent or supplementary prescribing.
3.  Prescribe safely, appropriately and cost effectively for both independent and supplementary prescribing.
4.  Understand the legislation relevant to the practice of independent and supplementary nurse prescribing.
5.  Understand and use sources of information, advice and decision support both in independent and supplementary prescribing practice.
6.  Understand the influences on independent and supplementary prescribing practice.
7.  Apply knowledge of drug actions in both independent and supplementary prescribing practice.
8.  Understand the roles and relationships of others involved in both independent and supplementary prescribing, supplying and administering medicines.
9.  Practise within a framework of professional accountability and responsibility in relation to both independent and supplementary nurse prescribing.
10. Draft a clinical management plan in conjunction with the independent prescriber.

Strategies used, for example, at De Montfort University (DMU) included:

⌘ Lectures and discussions to provide the knowledge to underpin practice and to promote student participation, sharing of views and exploration of attitudes.
⌘ Demonstration and experiential learning to promote the acquisition of practical skills.
⌘ Practice-based learning under the guidance of a medical supervisor to facilitate the application of theory to professional practice and the development of prescribing and related skills.
⌘ Teacher-led seminars to promote reflection, clinical learning and academic progress. Seminars also provided opportunities to address student issues.

- ⌘ Case analyses to promote reflection, critical analysis, decision-making and problem solving.
- ⌘ Role-modelling by teachers and medical supervisors to provide examples of good practice.
- ⌘ Student-led seminars to promote reflection, participation and independent study.
- ⌘ Computer-based learning/internet facilities and learning packages to promote flexibility and student-centred approaches.
- ⌘ Independent learning to develop the skills necessary for student-centred life-long learning.

Learning outcomes were required to be met in both theory and practice. The key person who was instrumental in achieving these learning outcomes in practice was the medical supervisor.

## Medical supervisors

Students on the extended independent prescribing course are usually expected to have, with support from their employer, their own medical supervisor. The prospective student nurse prescriber will tend to know her medical colleagues fairly well and will choose someone he/she can work with and who he/she expects to approach the task of supervision with some commitment.

The supervisor is asked to negotiate and clarify with the student how the supervision role will be fulfilled, to take account of respective commitments, best learning opportunities and other local considerations. The initial task of the supervisor is to assist the student in assessing their learning needs in relation to extended independent and/or supplementary prescribing within the practice setting.

The supervisor is encouraged to plan with the student the ways in which the identified learning needs can be met and implement the plan. This may include shadowing the medical supervisor or other medical prescribers, demonstration, discussion, observing the student, answering their questions, guiding and supporting them, pointing them to guidelines, protocols and other human or material resources.

At the end of the course the supervisor verifies the achievement of practice-based competence by completing the appropriate documentation.

## Preparation of medical supervisors

Universities offered their own methods of preparing medical supervisors for the task of supervising nurse-prescribing students. This was a challenging task because supervisors are busy people and they were often unable to attend study sessions in universities because of time or geographical constraints.

Information packages were sent out to medical practitioners, and in some cases these were the only form of preparation offered. The package would contain student course booklets and an introduction to some of the learning materials. The contents varied between universities. Mentors were encouraged to familiarise themselves with the contents prior to attending a two-hour preparatory workshop. A small number of workshops were held at different times with the hope of accommodating all mentors. Group preparation was the preferred option as this offered the opportunity to explore issues jointly and facilitated shared understanding and solutions as well as peer support. The course leader usually offered mentors who did not attend sessions a workplace visit; but again, this varied between universities and was limited by constraints such as time and geographical location.

## Support of medical supervisor

The course leader provides support and guidance regarding the course, any aspect of the supervision role, and deals with concerns regarding performance, attitude and motivation of the student.

Support for the supervisory role should have been obtained from the supervisor's employer or other colleagues if he or she was self-employed. The nature of the support required should have been negotiated prior to the start of the course. Inevitably, there were cases where this was not done until the supervisor had realised just how much of a commitment he or she had consented to and sometimes this lack of forward planning had a detrimental effect on the student and the supervisor.

Peer support from colleagues who had previously fulfilled the supervisory role could assist in role clarification, problem sharing and solving, sharing examples of good practice or pragmatic approaches to the role, and were utilised by many universities as a method of support.

## Supervision in practice

Twelve days or seventy-two hours practice learning is a considerable time commitment but, if used sensibly and creatively, offers student nurse prescribers the ideal opportunity to meet their learning needs in the practice situation. The seventy-two hours would encompass, for example, time spent in any useful learning experience which would help the student to meet the learning outcomes of the course. He or she might, for instance, spend two hours with the community pharmacist discussing dispensing issues, or the student might need to spend a morning with the tissue viability nurse discussing wound care issues. Time with other doctors would also give the student the opportunity to observe different consultation styles.

The theory to practice gap has long been recognised in nurse training, and what happens in clinical situations rarely mirrors the textbook scenario (Rolfe, 1996). The extended independent nurse prescribing course successfully integrates theory learned in the classroom situation with issues faced in practice. The mentor is instrumental in facilitating this process.

## Selection criteria for medical supervisors

Selection criteria for medical mentors laid down by the Department of Health are as follows:

⌘ To normally have had at least three years medical, treatment and prescribing responsibility for a group of patients/clients in the relevant field of practice.
⌘ To work within a GP practice and either be vocationally trained or have a certificate of equivalent training from the joint committee for post-graduate training in general practice.
⌘ Be a specialist registrar, clinical assistant or consultant within an NHS trust or other NHS employer?
⌘ To have some experience or training in teaching and/or supervising in practice.

(www. doh.gov.nurseprescribing)

## Assessment components

The validating body, the ENB, set the assessment of courses. They recognised that competence in prescribing would need to be demonstrated by assessment of theory and practice. The following four assessment methods were designed to test knowledge, decision making and the application of theory to practice (Leung, 2002). The four methods were:

● review of portfolio or learning log
● objective structured clinical examination

- satisfactory period of practice experience
- written final examination.

Plans for assessment were validated by the ENB before courses were implemented. An example of the mode of assessment utilised by De Montfort University is included below.

⌘ Submissions of a portfolio of evidence which has been compiled during the course, including the following:

  - an assessment of learning needs and a plan of action
  - an attendance log
  - a prescribing log
  - a practice-based assessment of prescribing competence
  - four client specific reflective case studies of 500 words each.

⌘ Students were also required to sit a two-hour final written examination. This examination consisted of a half-hour short answer/multiple choice questionnaire and two case study scenario questions which had to be answered in essay format and demonstrate that the student had an understanding of the entire process of prescribing and decision making in his or her answer.

Objective structured clinical examination (OSCE): This mode of assessment was designed at De Montfort by using four stations, at each of which the student spent fifteen minutes and was asked to complete a decision-making task. The task might be to write a prescription, to deal with a professional dilemma, or to describe the sort of questions she might ask a patient when making an assessment or deciding on a diagnosis.

A practice-based assessment of prescribing competence was required as part of the portfolio and had to be signed by the medical supervisor to provide evidence that learning outcomes had been met in practice (DMU, 2003).

## Professional body recognition

The qualification gained upon successful completion of either of the nurse prescribing courses are recordable on the Nursing and Midwifery Council's professional register as an annotation to the initial registration of the nurse.

**Competencies required for nurses supplying and administering medicines under patient group directions.**

*Chapter 2* describes how patient group directions (PGDs) are written and used. It is important to remember that nurses who supply and administer medications under patient group directions must demonstrate the competencies and hold the qualifications described in the PGD. There is no specific length of time specified from when the nurse qualifies at level one until she begins administration and supply using a PGD. She could theoretically use a PGD the day after she qualifies and employers should be aware that the nurse should have demonstrated her competence in the particular area prior to extending her practice in this way. The nurse should also have awareness of the legal and management issues associated with patient group directions. A nurse supplying under a PGD who does not comply with these competencies would be in breach of the law. It is also important that those who are responsible for writing patient group directions are aware of the need to detail specifically the nurse competencies necessary to supply and administer safely the drug in question. It follows that the nurse responsible for input into the creation of a PGD must have an understanding of the competencies and qualifications necessary for safe practice in that particular area. Nurses are responsible for being aware of their own scope of safe practice and employers should be aware of training needs through personal development plans. These are discussed in more detail in *Chapter 4*.

## References

De Montfort University (2002) *Course Handbook. Extended Independent Prescribing by Nurses Midwives and Health Visitors*. De Montfort University, Leicester

De Montfort University (2003) *Course Handbook: Extended Independent and Supplementary prescribing by Nurses, Midwives and Health Visitors*. De Montfort University, Leicester

Leung J (2002) The extended nurse-prescribing curriculum. *Br J Community Nurs* **7**(3): 143–7

Rolfe G (1996) *Closing the Theory to Practice Gap — a new paradigm for nursing*. Butterworth Heinmann, London

www.doh.gov.uk/nurseprescribing (accessed 21 April 2003)

# 4

## How does the nurse prescriber maintain competence?

The nurse prescriber will need to maintain competence in prescribing practice after qualification; indeed, it is his or her duty to do so (NMC, 2002). Reflection in and on experience (Schon, 1987) will help to develop practice and allow the nurse to develop from a competent, to an expert practioner (Benner, 1984). However, the nurse will also need support from other members of the team to develop his or her knowledge base, and confidence. Knowledge from updated information sources will be needed to develop competence. The employer, through the clinical governance framework, also has a responsibility to ensure that the nurse maintains her competence to prescribe so the issue can be seen as a joint responsibility between nurse and employer (Basford, 2003). Support will need to be consistent, timely and easily accessible. This is particularly crucial for the newly qualified prescriber, who will experience a delay between completing the course and being able to prescribe. Some delay is inevitable because of the time needed to annotate prescribing status on the NMC register, changing the job description and ordering and awaiting delivery of the prescription pad. This delay in starting to prescribe was, for some nurses in modes one and two of health visitor and district nurse prescribing, perceived as a barrier to prescribing (Basford, 2003; Otway, 2002). The delay represented an interruption in the educational process between learning in theory and prescribing in practice. The extended prescribing course is constructed differently, integrating theory and practice throughout the duration of the course. Local experience of early cohorts suggests that delay in getting started with prescribing will similarly be a difficult time for newly qualified prescribers.

### Information support

It is important to acknowledge that the activity of prescribing is one where the prescriber needs access to relevant, up-to-date and evidence-based information in the workplace. Every HV or DN prescriber is issued with a current edition of the *Nurse Prescribers' Formulary* (*NPF*). Every extended independent or supplementary prescriber is issued with the current edition of the *British National Formulary* (*BNF*) and all nurse prescribers receive the Drug Tariff every six months. However, to ensure that practice is evidence-based, it is also essential for the prescriber to have access to information from more up-to-date sources, for example, data bases such as the on-line version of the *BNF* as well as CINAHL, Bandolier and from web sites such as 'Nurse Prescriber' and 'The National Prescribing Centre' (a list of useful websites is listed in the references). In a study previously undertaken by the author (Otway, 2002), it was discovered that at the time of the study only 20% of nurses had access to the internet in their workplace. At the time of writing there is anecdotal evidence to support the fact that there has been a marked increase in that figure. The information strategy document (DoH, 2001a) supports the view that all health professionals should have access to the internet in their workplace, setting actions to ensure that this becomes a reality.

## Books and journals

The problem for many professional nurses is that having left university, they no longer have access to the academic library or to the array of professional journals published. Many nurses independently subscribe to one or two professional journals and if they are fortunate they are provided with access to one or two more in their workplace. It was found that nurses tended to read journals related to their own area of practice more commonly than generic nursing journals, and that most nurses read at least one journal on a regular basis although access was limited unless they bought the journal themselves (Otway, 2002). Prescribing information is best accessed through a journal which deals specifically with prescribing issues and could be made available in the workplace to ensure that all nurse prescribers have access. An example would be *Nurse Prescriber*, which was launched in February 2003.

## Newsletter

One way of helping nurse prescribers to keep updated is by local organisations producing a newsletter. It was found that this method of information dispersal was utilised well by nurse prescribers in two areas where research was undertaken (Basford, 2003; Otway, 2002). Leicestershire and Rutland NHS Trust was one of these areas. The newsletter was found to be a key factor in the successful dissemination of information and one, which has been used in many other areas. In the future this means of information dissemination can be used, either in the hard copy format or in the electronic version.

## Team or peer support

Isolation in practice was not found to be conducive to expanding the prescribing role or to creating confidence (Otway, 2001). Nurse prescribers need access to supportive peer groups of other nurse prescribers (Humphries and Green, 2000) and they also should have access to clinical supervision on a regular basis. Extended nurse prescribers are likely to be working in isolation, particularly in the early phase of development of extended nurse prescribing, due to the difficulty clinical areas have in releasing several members of staff at one time for training. It is therefore even more important to maintain contact via peer support networks and information support systems. There needs to be recognition of these needs from managers and an acknowledgment that protected time to keep updated and supported is necessary.

## Clinical governance

Nurse prescribing should take place within a framework of clinical governance (DoH, 2002) and this will help to support the nurse prescriber in the following ways.

### Clinical supervision

*Clinical supervision is a term used to describe a formal process of professional support and learning which enables individual practitioners to develop knowledge and competence, assume responsibility for their own practice and enhance consumer protection and safety of care in complex clinical situations. It is central to the process of learning, to the expansion of the scope of practice and should be seen as a means of encouraging assessment, analytical and reflective skills.*

(DoH, 1993)

This definition of clinical supervision, written at the time of the initial implementation of nurse prescribing, indicates how clinical supervision should be seen as an essential part of the process and development of the nurse prescribing initiative. It has been used in many areas but, unfortunately, tends to be neglected when practioners are busy or short-staffed (Otway, 2002). Clinical supervision is an essential ingredient for improving morale and for supporting staff through the change process (Bassett, 1999). Clinical supervision sessions between doctors, nurse prescribers and pharmacists have the potential for developing very safe and confident prescribing practice (DoH, 2002). In the future, the inclusion of other health professionals who have prescribing responsibilities would inevitably extend the benefits and ensure that clinical supervision and nurse prescribing go hand in hand to affect excellence in patient care.

## Personal development plans or appraisal systems

The *NHS Plan* (DoH, 2000) stated that systems of personal development planning (PDP) should be in place for every nurse. This was reiterated by the Government's plan for lifelong learning for the health service (DoH, 2001b). Anecdotal evidence suggests that although the appraisal system has been used in NHS organisations for some time, it has not been used consistently or regularly and has not always included action planning for future development of the employee. A recent survey (Leiffer, 2002) indicated that only 51% of participants, who were *Nursing Standard* readers, had a personal development plan in place; although 75% indicated that they had participated in an appraisal type interview with their manager in the preceding year. The PDP should set short, medium and long-term goals and include criteria for measuring whether goals have been achieved. The nurse also needs to receive formal feedback from his or her employer so that practice can be developed to meet the needs of the organisation and, ultimately, the needs of the client group as well as meeting the career aspirations of the nurse. Personal development planning should theoretically be an ongoing process starting with an assessment. Having formulated an action plan, the employer and the nurse should meet at regular intervals to reappraise progress and set more goals. In practice, the formal part of this process should happen once a year and the plan should be reviewed at least six-monthly to ensure that goals are met.

Personal development planning is particularly important when the nurse is extending his or her role, this applies to the nurse prescribing role. The National Prescribing Centre (NPC) have developed a 'competency framework' (NPC, 2001), which can be used alongside the PDP. This framework provides an outline of the competencies that nurse prescribers need to develop, to be safe, effective prescribers.

Nurse prescribers are encouraged to ask for a personal development plan if consistent systems are not already in place and are reminded to ensure that their new prescribing status is included in a revised job description, which should be rewritten before they commence prescribing.

**Clinical audit**

Clinical audit has been defined as:

> *The systematic and critical analysis of the quality of clinical care,*
> *including the procedures used for diagnosis, treatment and care,*
> *the associated use of resources and the resulting outcome and*
> *quality of life for the patient.*

(DoH, 1989)

Clinical audit can be utilised to inform prescribing practice. It is an ideal procedure for use with nurse prescribing because it enables prescribing to be analysed objectively as a specific area of practice (Humphries and Green, 2002) (*Figure 4.1*). Prescribing can be analysed from a financial as well as a clinical effectiveness point of view, and clinical audit will help to inform nurses about the appropriateness of their prescribing practice.

The audit cycle can be adapted for a prescribing audit as follows:

| | |
|---|---|
| I Identify a topic | This may, for example, be a type of dressing which recent published evidence may have shown to be more cost and clinically effective than another. |
| 2 Set criteria and standard | The criteria may be that type A dressing should be used on all patients with a leg ulcer. |
| 3 Collect data | The nursing team may decide to collect data from nursing records from one month, or a year to find out how many times the preferred dressing is prescribed as opposed to other types. |
| 4 Compare results with criteria | Compare results with criteria and standards. Results will be compared with the criteria |
| 5. Set an action plan only use the preferred dressing | For instance, this may be to decide to except in certain circumstances (eg. allergy) |
| 6 Re-audit | Re-audit may be done six months later to ensure that recommended change has been effective |

**Figure 4.1: Steps to prescribing audit**

## Research

Evidence-based practice has been defined as:

*An approach to decision making in which the clinician uses the best evidence available, in consultation with the patient, to decide upon the option which suits the patient best.*

Muir Gray, 1997

There has been much debate (le May, 2003) about what the evidence is and a hierarchy of evidence has been formulated (Long, 1996) which ranks evidence from research at the highest level. Much of the evidence base which informs prescribing practice is derived from quantitative data. However, the qualitative type of evidence is useful for examining the perceptions and experiences of patients and this type of research has gained in popularity.

Nurse prescribers will need to be able to access the evidence, appraise it and apply their knowledge to practice. These skills are an essential part of prescribing practice and are revised as part of the extended nurse-prescribing course.

## The National Prescribing Centre (NPC)

The NPC is a multidisciplinary National Health Service (NHS) organisation, funded by the Department of Health (DoH). Its aim is to facilitate the promotion of high quality, cost effective prescribing and medicines management through a co-ordinated and prioritised programme of activities, aimed at supporting all relevant professionals and senior managers working in the modern NHS.

The NPC has been involved in supporting nurse prescribers since 1998 and has a website containing useful information and downloadable documents, such as the *Signposts for Prescribing Nurses* which is also provided as a CD-Rom for extended nurse prescribing students. They also produce prescribing fact sheets and bulletins about particular conditions which nurses can treat in both hard copy and downloadable format. Details of their website can be found in the references section.

## The prescription pricing authority (PPA)

The PPA is an independent special health authority within the National Health Service. It has a wide number of functions, which it undertakes on behalf of the Secretary of State for Health. These include checking and pricing prescriptions and calculating reimbursements to dispensing contractors. It also analyses costs and prescribing trends. It compiles and publishes the Drug Tariff on a monthly basis and maintains the largest drug database in Europe.

Nurse prescribers working in primary care are required to inform the PPA of their prescribing details upon qualification, and are also required to keep the PPA updated on any changes of personal or prescribing details. The PPA passes on these details electronically to allow the printing of prescriptions upon request from the nurse prescriber's employer.

The prescription pricing authority (PPA) produces prescribing analysis and cost tabulation (PACT) data for individual GP prescribing practices. Nurses, prescribing within GP practices, should be able to access their own prescribing details with the help of the practice pharmacy advisor and this information can be used to analyse and inform individual prescribing practice. At an organisational level, PACT information is used to monitor and control prescribing costs and to set prescribing budgets (Lovejoy and Savage, 2001). This information should be utilised effectively by the nurse prescriber within the prescribing team to develop prescribing practice.

## References

Bassett C (1999) *Clinical Supervision: A guide for implementation*. NT Books, London

Basford L (2003) Maintaining nurse prescribing competence: Experience and challenges. *Nurse Prescribing* 1(1): 40–5

Benner P (1984) *From Novice to Expert: Excellence and Power in Clinical Nursing Practice*. Addison Wesley, Boston

Department of Health (1989) *Working for patients: The Health Service: Caring for the 1990s*. HMSO, London

Department of Health (1993) *A Vision for the future: The Nursing, Midwifery and Health Visiting contribution to Health and Healthcare*. HMSO, London

Department of Health (2001a) *Building the information core implementing the NHS plan*. DoH, London

Department of Health (2001b) *Working together learning together. A framework for lifelong learning in the NHS*. DoH, London

Department of Health (2002) *Extended independent nurse prescribing within the NHS in England: An implementation guide*. DoH, London

Humphries JL, Green J (2000) Nurse prescribers: infrastructures needed to support their role. *Nurs Standard* **14**(48): 35–9

Humphries JL, Green J (2002) *Nurse prescribing*. 2nd edn. Palgrave, Hampshire and New York

Leiffer (2002) Do you have a plan? *Nurs Standard* **16**(41): 15–17

le May Andree (2003) *Evidence Based Practice*. Nursing Times Clinical monographs No1, Emap Healthcare, London

Long A (1996) Health services research — a radical approach to cross the healthcare divide? In: Baker M, Kirk S eds. *Evidence Evaluation and Effectiveness*. Radcliffe Medical Press, Oxford

Lovejoy A, Savage I (2001) Prescribing analysis and cost tabulation (PACT) data: an introduction. *Br J Community Nurs* **6**(2): 62–7

Muir Gray J (1997) *Evidence-based Healthcare: How to make health policy and management decisions*. Churchill Livingstone, Edinburgh

National Prescribing Centre (2001) *Maintaining Competency in Prescribing: An outline framework to support nurse prescribers*. NPC, Liverpool

National Prescribing Centre: Online at: http://www.npc.ppa.nhs.uk

Nursing and Midwifery Council (2002) *Code of Professional Conduct*. NMC, London

Otway C (2001) Informal peer support: a key to success for nurse prescribers. *Br J Community Nurs* **6**(11): 586–91

Otway C (2002) The development needs of nurse prescribers. *Nurs Standard* **16**(18): 33–8

Schon D (1987) *Educating the Reflective Practitioner*. Jossey Bass, San Francisco and London

# 5

## The responsibilities of prescribing

Responsibility in nursing practice is something which nurses accept when they commence nurse training. The level of responsibility steadily increases as they increase their level and breadth of practice. Nurses are continually required to account for the decisions they make and there are times when responsibility weighs heavily upon them. The following definition of professional accountability is taken from the NMC guide for students of nursing and midwifery (2002):

> *Professional accountability involves weighing up the interests of patients, using your professional judgement and skill to make a decision and enabling you to account for the decision you make.*

It is important that at each juncture, prior to moving into a new area of practice, the nurse stops and reappraises that responsibility. A degree of self-awareness is necessary at this point as well as an honest appraisal of existing skills and knowledge. This is particularly important when it comes to prescribing because, unless the nurse is competent clinically, it may be that further training is indicated prior to undertaking the prescribing course. The prescribing course does not teach clinical skills, it prepares nurses for the prescribing role by teaching the principles and practice of prescribing. It also improves the consultation and diagnostic skills of the nurse so that safe prescribing decisions are made. Nurses increasingly recognise that their responsibility for direct care puts them in the decision makers role (Miers, 1990).

Some nurses may never be willing to take on the prescribing role because they do not have the competence or capability to prescribe (Basford and Bowskill, 2002). This is both acceptable and understandable given the degree of responsibility required. Other nurses, who have prescribing qualifications, opt not to prescribe in circumstances where the logistics of completing the task safely are hindered; for instance, where access to records is problematic (Dion, 2002). Many more nurses have, and will continue to take on prescribing responsibilities for the benefit of patient care, after they have completed the required educational preparation. It could be agreed that an extension of prescribing power without the accompanying and essential knowledge base would, indeed, be very dangerous for patients. However, nurses have a sound code of professional practice upon which to base their decisions. It could be argued that any nursing procedure or intervention could be just as potentially dangerous if approached without the necessary skills or knowledge, as prescribing incorrectly could be. Although potential nurse prescribers need to be aware of their responsibility, balanced against their overall responsibility to patients on a daily basis, particularly in the administration of medicines, they can feel confident that as long as they practice thoughtfully and reflectively, they can safely develop prescribing skills.

The prescriber is responsible for the prescription he or she signs (DoH, 2002). Until nurses become qualified prescribers they have not, in law, been responsible for prescribing, but they have always been responsible for administration of medicines and dressings. Nurses, prior to becoming prescribers, will have been aware of the drugs or medications they have been administering. This has always been a part of core nursing practice:

> *The administration of medicines is an important aspect of the professional practice of persons whose names are on the councils' register. It is not solely a mechanistic task to be performed in strict compliance with the written prescription of the medical practitioner, it requires thought and the exercise of professional judgement.*
>
> (NMC 2002)

Nurses have, in the past, been held legally accountable for administering incorrect dosages of medication and shared in accountability, even when the incorrect administration has been due to a doctor's prescribing error (Dimond, 1995). They may also have been actively involved in advising patients on the use of over the counter medications: in this context they would have been seen to be undertaking a form of prescribing according to definition opposite.

Many nurses would say that, according to this definition, they have been prescribing for years, or finding strategies to circumvent the inconvenience of not being legally allowed to prescribe (Jones, 1999). They have been advising doctors of what to write on drug charts or prescriptions, often writing prescriptions or printing them off the practice computer and asking a doctor to sign the prescription. Consequently, some nurses feel that they are already competent in many elements of the required learning outcomes of the extended prescribing course. They often feel that they have adequately covered accountability, legal and ethical aspects of nursing on previous courses. This is reassuring because nurses should be well aware of the law and how it affects their practice. However, prior to starting, it is important to understand and explore the particular issues regarding prescribing practice legally, in order to have a full appreciation of the responsibility held in law. We are all expected to know the law; ignorance of the law is no defence (Tingle, 1990). However much knowledge the nurse has before embarking on the prescribing course, he or she will never have been accountable before for the content of a prescription. Evidence shows that nurses become very anxious and acutely aware of their accountability when they are actually qualified as prescribers and have to sign their first few prescriptions (Luker *et al*, 1998; Lowe and Hurst, 2002).

> **Prescribe**: in the legal sense, as used in the Medicines Act:
> i. To order in writing the supply of a prescription only medicine for a named patient;
> But commonly used in the extended sense of:
> ii to authorise by means of an NHS prescription the supply of any medicine(not just a prescription only medicine) at public expense.
> And occasionally
> iii to advise a patient on suitable care or medication (including medicine which may be bought over the counter.
> (DoH, 1999).

There are four arenas of accountability (Dimond, 1995):

| | |
|---|---|
| ⌘ Criminal law | Accountable to the court |
| ⌘ Civil law | Accountable to the court |
| ⌘ Professional accountability | Accountable to the NMC |
| ⌘ Employment accountability | Accountable to the employer |

Nurses may be called to account in any or all of these arenas, but the one not listed above, which will be of constant significance to the nurse will be the moral dimension of accountability to the self, in terms of professional competence and skill (Dimond, 1995). This one, of course, can never be quantified but it is one arena, which should not be forgotten. Indeed, to the conscientious nurse this is one arena that is never forgotten and can be the cause of a lot of stress and insomnia!

There are three areas of conduct (Preece, 2002) for which nurses are accountable. These are

- personal conduct
- professional conduct
- professional practice.

Each of these areas of conduct may fall into any of the four arenas of accountability.

## Criminal law

The laws, which particularly relate to prescribing, are:

⌘ The Medicines Act (1968) which restricts the prescribing of prescription only medicines to appropriate practitioners defined in the act as registered medical practitioners, registered dentists and registered veterinary practitioners, and the The Medicinal Products: Prescription by Nurses Act (1992) and subsequent legislation under that act permits certain nurses to prescribe from a limited formulary.

These acts make any infringement a criminal offence. Nurse prescribers have to be sure that they remain within their scope of practice and the *Nurse Prescribers' Formulary* from which they are qualified to prescribe (Preece, 2002).

⌘ The Misuse of Drugs Act (1971) legislates for controls on drugs, which are considered to be dangerous, and the amendments to this act classify these drugs into Section 1, 2, 3, 4, and 5 drugs. The control of these drugs lies with the Home Office and the Medicines Control Agency. Nurses are not currently able to prescribe any controlled drugs but the matter is currently under review.

## Civil law

The above laws are examples of statute law but much of healthcare law is derived from common or case law (Tingle, 1990). Civil courts deal mainly with negligence claims. In the case of health professionals, to prove negligence a claimant has to prove three things:

1 That a duty of care existed. This would mean that the claimant was actually a patient of the accused health professional.
2 That the duty of care had been breached.
3 That damage had been caused to the claimant.

The breach to the duty of care is judged by applying the Bolam test. The Bolam test is an example of case law, which was decided following a now famous case between Bolam and Friern Hospital (*Bolam* v *Friern Barnet*

*HMC* [1957]). The claimant, Bolam, accused a doctor of negligence. In a court of law it would be very difficult for the judge to decide whether a doctor had in fact been negligent, when the judge himself was not qualified to know what would actually constitute negligence in a complicated medical case. The principle therefore states that:

> *Where there is uncertainty the court will ask the opinion of a responsible body of medical men skilled in that particular art.*

A subsequent case, *Bolitho* v *Hackney* [1997] defined this test even further, highlighting that the responsible group of men, or the peer group who are consulted by the court, have to be responsible and not themselves using unacceptable practice.

## Employment accountablity

This type of accountability relates to job descriptions, which have to change in order for the nurse to be able to prescribe and policies and procedures which nurses are expected to adhere to when employed by a particular trust. Stepping outside of these boundaries might result in disciplinary action. It is quite reasonable for the employer to ask staff to adhere to guidelines because the employer is vicariously liable for the actions of an employee. If an employee is sued, the employer will, under vicarious liability, pay the costs of the damage. If the employee was not following the accepted guidelines or in breach of their job description, the employer could sue the employee for damages.

## Professional accountability

All nurses are accountable to the Nursing and Midwifery Council (NMC). Nursing qualifications have to be registered with the council in order for nurses to practice. Nurse prescribers have the register annotated with their qualifications and are not legally allowed to prescribe until they receive notification from the NMC. Pharmacists can check on the NMC voicemessaging service to find out whether a nurse is qualified as a prescriber before they dispense a prescription. Registration depends on the NMC and can be withdrawn in cases of misconduct.

The following scenarios illustrate some of the areas of responsibility that nurse prescribers may face on a daily basis. They highlight how the legal framework can be applied in practice. This section does not give answers, it raises questions for discussion.

There are some key documents which are helpful when considering these scenarios, and which should be available for consultation by the nurse prescriber. These are:

- ⌘ Nursing and Midwifery Council (2002) *Code of professional conduct.* NMC, London
- ⌘ United Kingdom Central Council for Nursing Midwifery and Health Visiting (1992) *Scope of Professional Practice.* UKCC, London
- ⌘ Nursing and Midwifery Council (2002) *Guidelines for the administration of medicines.* NMC, London
- ⌘ United Kingdom Central Council for Nursing Midwifery and Health Visiting (2001) *Covert administration of medicines.* UKCC, London

## Scenario one

Mrs Jones attends the doctor's surgery with her baby daughter aged three months. She gives verbal consent to the administration of a vaccine for her baby and then asks the nurse prescriber for a prescription for paracetamol oral suspension. The mother says that due to financial problems she is unable to purchase paracetamol today. The baby developed mild pyrexia and was fretful after the first vaccination and the mother is concerned that this may happen again.

The dilemma is that the vaccine has been given and may induce pyrexia during the next twenty-four to forty-eight hours (*BNF* 43). This is considered to be a common and normal reaction and can be safely treated with paracetamol. Paracetamol oral suspension can be bought over the counter and the nurse suggests this to the mother. The unwritten practice policy states that paracetamol should not be prescribed routinely.

What would your prescribing decision be?

### Points for discussion

Key point from the Nursing and Midwifery Council's *Code of Conduct*:

1 As a registered nurse, midwife or health visitor you must respect the patient or client as an individual.

- ❖ The baby is your patient and her mother is the carer.
- ❖ The mother is creating pressure for you to prescribe.
- ❖ The unwritten practice policy is another source of pressure — should

this policy be written and communicated to all carers to take some of the pressure off the prescriber?
* Is the practice policy a good and safe one?
* If the baby does not have paracetamol what is the outcome likely to be?

## Scenario two

You decide to write a prescription at the vaccination clinic for paracetamol for one client. You make this decision on an individual basis for one patient because you believe that on this occasion, if you did not prescribe, then the child would not receive the treatment you have recommended, or she might be likely to be given another product which might be unsafe. If she developed post immunisation pyrexia she would suffer pain discomfort as a result and so, on balance of risk, you make the decision that a prescription for paracetamol is the best and safest option in this case. The mother and child leave the room with the prescription. The next client sees the prescription and also asks for a prescription for paracetamol for her baby and she says that she saw you issue one to the last patient and so feels that she is also entitled to a free prescription for her child.

How do you respond?

## Points for discussion

Key point from the Nursing and Midwifery Council's *Code of Conduct*:

5  As a registered nurse or midwife you must respect confidential information.

and,

1  As a registered nurse, midwife or health visitor you must respect the patient or client as an individual.

The dilemma is that you cannot share the information you had about patient A with patient B. You must offer both individualised treatment but that does not always result in the same outcome.

## Scenario three

A client attends your skin clinic with her two children. She says that she has been using the cream prescribed for her son on her daughter's rash, which she presumes to be the same as the rash her son has which was diagnosed as eczema.

The dilemma here is that the client is using an item on one child, which has been prescribed for another child. The cream prescribed can be bought over the counter but the mother is saving time and money in using cream prescribed for someone else.

### Points for discussion

Key point from the Nursing and Midwifery Council's *Code of Conduct*:

1   As a registered nurse, midwife or health visitor you must respect the patient or client as an individual.

8   As a registered nurse you must act to identify and minimise the risk to patients and clients.

❖   The patients are the children who should both be provided with individual care relating to individual diagnoses.

❖   Using cream prescribed for one child to both children gives misleading information to the prescriber about the extent of the problem in both cases.

## Scenario four

An elderly lady asks you how she can get her husband to take his medications, she wants to know if she can open the capsules and conceal the contents in his food. He is refusing treatment but the lady wants him to take the tablets, which you have prescribed.

The dilemma here is relating to the covert administration of medicines. Consent to treatment applies equally to all patients and you should assume that every patient is legally competent unless otherwise assessed by a suitably qualified practitioner.

The second dilemma is that in opening the capsules and altering the formulation you may be prescribing out of the product licence.

## Points for discussion

Key point from the Nursing and Midwifery Council's *Code of Conduct*:

3  As a registered nurse, midwife or health visitor you must obtain consent before you give any treatment or care.

## Scenario five

A friendly and helpful pharmaceutical company representative offers you a weekend at a health spa in return for consenting to prescribe ten new wound care products made by his company.

The dilemma here is that you would love to go to the health spa for the weekend but you are also aware that there is 'no such thing as a free lunch'. The wound care products are new and you are unaware of their efficacy as there has been only one small scale study done, which was commissioned by the pharmaceutical company.

## Points for discussion

Key point from the Nursing and Midwifery Council's *Code of Conduct*:

7  As a registered nurse, midwife or health visitor, you must be trustworthy.

1  As a registered nurse, midwife or health visitor you must respect the patient or client as an individual.

❖  The pharmaceutical representative is offering more to you than is acceptable according to his code of practice.
❖  The wound care products are new so evidence is limited.
❖  Each patient should be prescribed individual care — not prescribe a new dressing just because you want to win your free weekend.

## Scenario six

A gentleman attends your minor ailment session. He is a little abrupt and says he is in a hurry. He would like a prescription for some antibiotics to take for his sore throat. He woke up with the sore throat this morning but wants to get rid of it as he has an important weekend conference coming up. He has been prescribed antibiotics for this problem before and it worked.

The dilemma here is that this could well be a viral infection and antibiotics will have no effect.

You are aware of the antimicrobial policy in the trust which, if followed, would not allow you to prescribe antibiotics.

**Points for discussion**

Key point from the Nursing and Midwifery Council's *Code of Conduct*:

1   As a registered nurse, midwife or health visitor you must respect the patient or client as an individual.

4   As a registered nurse you must co-operate with others in the team.

❖  The patient in this case really needs to understand why he does not require antibiotics but he is possibly not very receptive today.
❖  An easy option might be to prescribe, but would this be a wise option?

**References**

Basford L, Bowskill D (2002) Celebrating the past, challenging the future of nurse prescribing. In: *Topics in Nurse Prescribing,* volume 1 (*British Journal of Community Nursing* monograph). Quay Books, MA Healthcare Limited, Salisbury

*Bolam v Friern Barnet HMC* [1957] 1 All ER 118 25
*Bolitho v City and Hackney HA* [1997] 3 WLR 115 25
British National Formulary 43 (2002) *British National Formulary* Section 14. British Medical Association, Royal pharmaceutical Society of Great Britain, London
Department of Health (1999) Review of Prescribing, Supply and Administration Final Report (Crown 2). HMSO, London.
Department of Health (2002) *Extending Independent Nurse Prescribing within the NHS in England:A guide for implementation*. Crown copyright. Department of Health Publications. London
Dimond B (1995) *Legal Aspects of Nursing*. 2nd edn. Prentice Hall, Europe

Dion X (2002) Record keeping and nurse prescribing — an issue of concern? In: *Topics in Nurse Prescribing*, volume 1 *(British Journal of Community Nursing* monograph). Quay Books, MA Healthcare Limited, Salisbury

Nursing and Midwifery Council (2002) *Guidelines for the administration of medicines*. Online at: http://www.nmc-uk.org (accessed 16/4/03)

Jones M (1999) *Nurse Prescribing: Politics to practice*. Ballière Tindall, Royal College of Nursing, London

Lowe L, Hurst R (2002) Nurse prescribing: The reality. In: Humphries J, Green J, *Nurse Prescribing*. 2nd edn. Palgrave, London

Luker K, Hogg C, Austin l, Ferguson B, Smith K (1998) Decision making: The context of nurse prescribing. *J Adv Nurs* **27**: 657–65

Miers M (1990) Developing skills in decision making. *Nurs Times* **86**(30):

Nursing and Midwifery Council (2002) *A guide for students of nursing and midwifery*. NMC, London

Preece S (2002) Nurse prescribing: Accountability and legal issues. In: Humphries J, Green J *Nurse prescribing*. 2nd edn. Palgrave, London

Tingle J (1990) Making the law. *Nurs Times* **87**(31): 52–3

# 6

## The art and science of prescribing

The term prescribe is defined as:

⌘ To order in writing the supply of a prescription only medicine (POM) for a named patient.
⌘ To authorise by means of an NHS prescription the supply of any medicine at public expense.
⌘ To advise a patient on suitable care or medication which may be purchased over the counter (OTC) without a written order (DoH, 1999).

As this definition describes, to prescribe does not always involve writing a prescription. Many nurses will have, following the latter part of this definition, claim to have been prescribing for years. Indeed, there will be many times where the qualified independent or supplementary nurse prescriber will decide not to prescribe at all. However, after qualifying as a nurse prescriber of any type, the nurse will inevitably be making prescribing decisions for the rest of his or her working life. The decision-making process surrounding prescribing is a complex one and, once learned, will become an implicit part of the nurse's knowledge, skills and attitude base.

The first step in the prescribing process is to consult with the patient, accurately assess the patient's condition and arrive at a diagnosis. Nurses may learn to consult using a variety of methods. They may enter a nurse prescribing course feeling that they already have refined and advanced diagnostic and/or assessment skills and feel affronted that the course will attempt to teach them what they have been practising for many years. Attempting effectively to teach students from a variety of clinical backgrounds and types of experience is challenging.

There are many ways of meeting this challenge and one interesting model has been developed at Leicester University. A teaching package has been adapted for nurses (CAIIN, Redsell, 2002) from a package designed for GP trainees (Fraser, 1994), which aims to improve consultation skills. This framework is useful for all prescribers with varying lengths and types of experience because it helps to build on and improve existing skills by analysing current performance and giving strategies or suggestions for improvement. CAIIN is taught by a GP who has used the tool in his own practice. It is produced as a framework which gives students the opportunity to observe other colleagues in practice and identify weaker areas of practice which might need to be improved.

During the consultation, the nurse will gather all the relevant information needed and will attempt to problem solve by arriving at an assessment conclusion or diagnosis. During this process, the nurse will be aware of her own scope of practice (UKCC, 1992) and will refer to a medical colleague if the case falls outside of those boundaries.

Once a decision has been made about whether a prescribable item is indicated, the nurse will need to decide whether or not a prescription is needed. Prescriptions are issued for a variety of reasons and not all prescribing achieves a successful outcome (NPC, 2002). Prescribers are affected by many outside influences and need to be aware of those issues during the decision-making process. Patients can be very demanding and insist that they are prescribed what they perceive to be the best treatment for themselves (some examples have been described in *Chapter 5*). Patient centredness does not, of course, mean that the prescriber must compromise his or her professional decision making in order to please the patient. A concordant model of prescribing will be adopted which identifies the patient and nurse in an equal partnership. In signing a prescription the prescriber takes full accountability for his or her actions. The patient's knowledge may well be based on incorrect or limited information and the prescriber has to sometimes re-educate the patient during the consultation. An example might be the patient who demands an antibiotic for a viral infection. The issues are complex and affect far more than the direct patient/nurse relationship. The challenges faced by the prescriber in explaining antimicrobial resistance in the course of a relatively short consultation are immense.

The nurse is advised to use a concordant model of care in order to achieve a successful prescribing outcome. Concordance means that the patient and the nurse are equal in the decision-making process and there is an exchange of information and co-operation between the two. The patient is fully aware of the diagnosis and the aim of treatment. It logically follows that he or she will be more likely to tolerate and co-operate with treatment and also be more likely to return to the prescriber if the prescribed treatment does not help to treat the condition effectively, or, if it causes unwanted side-effects or adverse reactions.

Prescribable items are classified into three types by the Medicines Act 1968:

- ⌘ Prescription only medicines (POMs)
- ⌘ Pharmacy medicines (P medicines)
- ⌘ Over the counter medicines (OTC)

The nurse prescriber may write a prescription for any of these three types of items. However, it will depend on whether or not the item needed by the patient is included in the *Nurse Prescribers' Formulary,* from which the nurse is qualified to prescribe or is included in the patient's clinical management plan.

## Prescriptions

NHS prescriptions are written on either an FP10P or on a patient drug chart or hospital out-patient prescription.

Different types of prescribers use different versions of the standard FP10. Each version is a different colour, both types of nurse prescribers currently prescribe on a lilac coloured pad, which helps the dispenser and the PPA to identify the prescriber. The different versions also have different codes:

❖ Community nurse prescribers use the FP10P. This is printed with information to denote the type of prescriber, eg. district nurse or health visitor prescriber followed by their name and NMC PIN number.
❖ Extended independent nurse prescriber, supplementary prescriber name and NMC PIN number.
❖ Hospital nurse prescribers use the FP10HP and this form is stamped with extended nurse prescriber and their NMC PIN number.

It is important to remember that each primary care trust (PCT) has its own prescription pads. Prescribed items for each patient will be costed to the PCT prescribing budget where the patient's general practitioner resides, not where the patient resides, therefore the nurse needs to have permission from each PCT to prescribe for patients belonging to the PCT and will be issued with PCT prescription pads after permission to prescribe has been considered. Unfortunately, this might mean that a nurse who works across several PCT areas will need to carry several prescription pads. She will also need to check in patient's records, which patient belongs to which PCT before writing the prescription. The nurse prescriber will also need to add the patient's practice code to the prescription.

## Role of the prescription pricing authority (PPA)

The PPA has to be notified of the details of every primary care nurse prescriber before prescriptions can be ordered from the printer (Astron). The PPA will require details updating and nurses should remember to inform the PPA if they change name or move to a new post.

## Ordering prescription pads

Each trust will have a designated person who is responsible for ordering and distributing prescription pads. Prescribers should remember to order enough prescriptions to keep them supplied for practice, but should not order too many that they cannot store them safely. Each prescription has a serial number and these numbers should be recorded each time the nurse collects a new pad.

## Safekeeping of prescription pads

Prescribers are advised to keep prescription pads safely at all times. They are advised to take the same care of the prescription pad as they would of their own chequebook.

Prescriptions should never be presigned and should be kept either with the prescriber or locked away safely when not in use. Lost or stolen prescription pads, which fall into the wrong hands, could provide the means to obtain prescribable items for criminal purposes: it is imperative that pads are carefully handled.

## Lost or stolen prescription pads

If prescription pads are lost or stolen, their loss must be reported immediately to the prescribing lead nurse in the trust and to the nurse manager or whatever policy their own trust has in place. A security procedure is put in place to inform the police and all pharmacies in the area so that illegal prescriptions are not dispensed. If the nurse has accurately recorded serial numbers when she took delivery of her prescription pad, he or she can, in the event of the loss of a prescription pad, provide the police with exact details of which pads are missing. Blank prescriptions should never be pre-signed in case of theft or fraud.

## Practice codes

After the nurse has ensured that he or she is using the correct prescription pad the nurse needs to remember to enter the correct practice prescribing code in the appropriate box. (Practice nurses will have this code pre-printed on their prescriptions.) If this is not correctly completed then the prescription charges will not be charged to the correct budget or they may not be charged to any budget at all. This results in the prescription being returned to the prescriber or to the prescriber's employer at a later date for verification. The entire process may take six months or longer and causes administration problems, costing problems, as well as embarrassment for the prescriber concerned.

## Handwritten versus computer-generated prescriptions

Although computer issued prescriptions save time and reduce errors they are still not available for nurse prescribers at the time of writing. Unfortunately, practice appears to have overtaken technology, and nurses have recently been assured that development in this area is taking place. Hopefully, in the not too distant future, nurses will be able as their medical colleagues to print prescriptions from the practice computer. As many prescriptions are, and will continue to be, written in the home of the patient, or in the ward setting without the aid of a computer it will be, for the foreseeable future, essential for nurses to be competent in prescription writing.

Handwriting should be clear and legible. Pharmacists are not official interpreters but they are often expected to read correctly hastily written scripts. Not only is this inconsiderate on the part of the prescriber, it is also dangerous. However busy prescribers are, it is imperative that prescriptions are written clearly and carefully in order to avoid potentially fatal mistakes.

## Legal requirements

The following items must be legally included in any prescription.

- name of patient
- address
- age
- date of birth (this is a preferable requirement and becomes a legal requirement if the patient is under twelve years of age).

The prescription should be dated and signed by the prescriber. It must be remembered that the responsibility for the prescription rests with the person who signs the prescription.

## Items to be prescribed

Prescribable items should, wherever possible, be described by generic name. This ensures that the most cost effective and readily available product can be supplied as quickly as possible. Some items, for example family planning products, need to be prescribed by brand name because the generic name would not adequately describe the intention of the prescriber.

It is good practice to open the *NPF* to clarify details of amounts and dosages every time a prescription is written in order to ensure that errors do not occur. Nurses may well have been used to double-checking their administration of medicines and, if not, will have developed their own procedure for double-checking their own practice. When prescribing they will find that they are unlikely to be able physically to double check because they are alone in the home or clinic. They will need to develop their own method of writing and carefully double-checking prescribing details. Amounts should be written clearly and dosages should be stated. Abbreviations and Latin terminology should be avoided to ensure clarity and safety.

## Incorrectly written prescriptions

If prescriptions are incorrectly written or are incomplete the pharmacist should contact the prescriber and ask them to amend the prescription accordingly. It is important that the prescriber includes his or her contact telephone number on the prescription so he or she can be easily contacted.

## Adverse drug reaction reporting

All drugs are capable of causing unintended responses or adverse effects. It is impossible to be 100% sure that every possible ill effect is identified before a drug appears on the market (Prosser *et al*, 2000). The definition of an adverse drug reaction is as follows:

> *An unwanted or harmful reaction experienced following the administration of a drug or combination of drugs under normal conditions of use, and is suspected to be related to the medicine.*
> (MCA, 2002)

It is important that nurse prescribers are aware of the procedure to be followed in the case of an adverse drug reaction. Until recently, only medical independent prescribers were allowed to report adverse drug reactions, but since October 2002 the yellow card scheme operated by the Medicines Control Agency (MCA) has been extended to nurses, midwives and health visitors.

The yellow card scheme for spontaneous reporting of suspected adverse drug reactions was introduced in 1964 after the thalidomide tragedy highlighted the urgent need for routine post marketing surveillance of medicines.

Yellow cards are found at the back of the *British National Formulary*, the *Nurse Prescribers' Formulary* and the *Monthly Index of Medical Specialities Companion* (MIMS), and there is also an electronic version available which can be found online at: www.mca.gov.uk/yellowcard

Information to be included on the yellow card relates to:

- suspect drug
- suspect reaction
- patient details
- reporter details.

## References

Department of Health (1999) *Report of the Advisory Group on Nurse Prescribing.* Crown report. HMSO, London.

Department of Health (2002) *Extending Independent Nurse Prescribing within the NHS in England: An implementation guide.* Crown Copyright. Department of Health publications, London

Department of Health (2003) *Supplementary Prescribing by Nurses and Pharmacists within the NHS in England: An implementation guide.* Crown Copyright. Department of Health publications. London

Department of General Practice and Primary Healthcare (2002) *Consultation Assessment and Improvement Instrument for Nurses.* 1st edn. Department of General Practice and Primary Healthcare, University of Leicester

Fraser RC (1994) *Assessment of Consultation Competence. The Leicester Assessment Package.* 2nd edn. Macclefield. Glaxo Medical Fellowship

Medicines Control Agency (2002) *Extension of the Yellow Card Scheme to Nurse Reporters.* MCA, London

National Prescribing Centre (2002) Signposts for prescribing nurses — CD ROM. NPC, Liverpool

Prosser S, Worster B, Macgregor J, Dewar K, Runyard P, Fegan J (DATE) *Applied Pharmacology: An introduction to pathophysiology and drug management for nurses and healthcare professionals.* Mosby, London and New York, Philadelphia, St Louis, Sydney, Toronto

Redsell S, Hastings A, Cheater F, Fraser R (2003) Devising and establishing face and content validity of explicit criteria of consultation competence in UK primary care nurses. *Nurse Education Today* **23**(4): 299–306

United Kingdom Central Council for Nursing, Midwifery and Health Visiting (1992) *Scope of Professional Practice*. UKCC, London

# 7

# Roles and responsibilities

*All the world's a stage.*
*And all the men and women merely players:*
*They all have their exits and their entrances;*
*And one man in his time plays many parts.*

*(As You Like It*, II. vii. 139–143)

Shakespeare was relating to the seven ages of man when he wrote this well-known and often quoted stanza. It is quoted here to remind us how the nurse, as prescriber, may occupy many roles within the prescribing process, from assessment and diagnosis, supply and administration, through to prescribing.

Successful prescribing occurs within a team context, and the knowledge, skills and attitudes of the nurse prescriber will inevitably have an impact upon the rest of the team. A successful team is one that achieves its aim in the most efficient way and is ready to take on more challenging tasks (Adair, 1986). As an independent prescriber and possibly the only prescriber in the nursing team, the other nurse members may well see the nurse prescriber as the expert in prescribing and knowledge of medicines and other prescribable items, as well as knowledge about general prescribing issues. This can place increasing demands on the prescriber both in terms of sharing knowledge and expertise but also in managing their own role of prescriber.

*The expert must therefore have skills in human relations as well as*
*in his own field if he is to function usefully in a group where other*
*members are less skilled than he is.*

(Klein, 1956)

The prescriber will need to be aware of the demands that the role places on them within the team; be aware of their own professional boundaries and also be clear about their own accountability.

One of the difficulties in being the first nurse prescriber within a nursing team is coping with the perceptions of the other team members. There may be conflict due to professional jealousy (Skidmore, 2002), or unrealistic demands made by team members who expect the nurse prescriber to write prescriptions for every patient. The nurse can only prescribe for patients she has previously assessed (DoH, 2002) and will need to make it clear to other members of the team where the boundaries lie.

The role of the leader within the team is to help the team achieve its common task, to maintain it as a unit and to ensure that each individual contributes his best (Adair, 1986). The nurse prescriber, as leader, also has a responsibility to inspire and motivate other team members to improve the collective team achievement. The nurse prescriber needs to keep other non-prescribing team members aware of developments in prescribing (Humphries and Green, 2002). This is particularly important for the extended formulary prescriber who will have had the support of other team members to access the extended independent and supplementary course in the first place. The newly qualified prescriber can now play their part by supporting colleagues while they go for training. Subsequently, more patients can benefit and the team as a whole can maximise its effectiveness. This puts the role of the nurse prescriber in a very positive position both as expert, supporter and motivator. Lack of awareness of this responsibility on the part of the prescriber can be detrimental to the team and might deny others the benefit of the shared knowledge they would otherwise gain.

However, in the wider sense of the team, the nurse may well be seen as the novice. The nurse prescriber member of the primary healthcare team or the nurse member of the medical prescribing team within the acute setting can feel isolated, particularly if she is the first nurse to train as a prescriber, as inevitably some nurses will be. In reality, the nurse may or may not be a novice in terms of competence, knowledge and skill acquisition, but may initially be seen in those terms until she proves otherwise, to some of the more experienced medical prescribers. This apparent confusion of role identity will cause inevitable pressures for the nurse prescriber; but they are pressures which she will have learned to deal with throughout her nursing experience in other areas of practice.

The key to facilitating good relationships is to communicate effectively using all the previously learned communication skills as well as accessing newer methods such as fax and email. Although these methods are commonplace in industry and commerce they are still relatively new to many nurses. The essential communication skill in relation to prescribing is, of course, record keeping. All nurses are required to keep contemporaneous records, which are unambiguous and legible (NMC, 2002). This is the case in the area of prescribing but, unfortunately, the newer and easier methods of computerised prescribing are not currently available for the nurse prescriber to use. Nurses have been informed that work is currently underway to improve this situation and eagerly await this improvement. At the current time, the nurse has to write the prescription and record the details in the patient's record and in the medical record, along with other important details of the consultation. The nurse also needs to have access to the medical record before she prescribes so that she can ensure that she does not prescribe something which will adversely interact with currently prescribed medications. This is not so much a problem in the secondary care setting, where patient, nurse and doctor are all located in the same place. It can be difficult, however, for nurses working in primary care, particularly in rural areas where long distances exist between services. In the case of supplementary prescribing, there has to be even more co-operation and effective communication between the independent and the supplementary prescribers and, in the initial stages, effective and safe systems need to be constructed to ensure safe prescribing practice.

The role of the nurse prescriber in the team context, as defined by the National Prescribing Centre, states that the nurse:

⌘ Establishes relationships with colleagues based on understanding of, and respect for, each other's roles (NPC, 2002).

The rest of this chapter is devoted to describing some of the roles and functions of the less well known members of the prescribing team.

## Nurse prescribing lead

A senior nurse within each PCT or hospital trust with an enthusiasm and commitment to developing nurse prescribing will be identified to take the lead on nurse prescribing issues. Depending on the size of the trust, this may be a complete job role, but it will, more commonly, be part of a job role. The nurse lead will often have an advisory role within the trust at strategic level, and one of his or her responsibilities at field level will be to facilitate and co-ordinate support for nurse prescribers. There will be organisational issues, such as ordering and storage of prescription pads as well as arranging clinical supervision sessions and clinical updating. Nurse prescribers need to have a named nurse to contact in situations where support is needed on a one-to-one basis. The potential nurse prescriber will contact the lead nurse in the first instance, when he or she is considering applying for prescribing training. The lead nurse will help the potential prescriber to think through the issues around whether prescribing will be of benefit to the patients cared for, and will also discuss the issues with the nurse manager before signing the nomination form to apply to the local workforce confederation for funding for training. The lead nurse will also need to co-ordinate the distribution of new national initiatives or guidelines for prescribing practice and will need to feed information from the grass roots level through to regional and national nurse prescribing leads.

## Independent medical prescriber

This team member may be a junior houseman, registrar or consultant within the secondary care setting, and a general practitioner (GP) in primary care. He or she is a significant team member, particularly because of the prescribing role which he or she will always have held since qualifying as a doctor. As discussed earlier, the attitudes of doctors towards nurses prescribing are varied and attitudes will vary within one hospital department or one practice. The nurse prescriber has to work with all these members of staff regardless of their views. The most crucial significant role a medical practitioner can hold for the nurse prescriber is that of medical supervisor. This role has been discussed earlier but the role as a supporter of the nurse prescriber is, hopefully, one which will continue to be held in an informal way, long after the course has finished.

## Pharmaceutical representatives

Pharmaceutical representatives can be a useful source of information for nurse prescribers. They are mentioned here as indirect members of the nurse prescribing team. The impact of the pharmaceutical representative will depend very much on the attitude of the trust or the particular nursing team involved. Trusts have different collective attitudes to pharmaceutical representatives and may have policies in place regarding the access arrangements that representatives might have to nursing teams. These policies range from limited access to no access at all, and have often been created partly because of the time which could be potentially taken in seeing representatives and because of limiting nurses' access to information which is understandably biased. Nurse prescribers are taught to evaluate critically sources of information and are made aware of the influence of marketing by pharmaceutical companies. Large pharmaceutical companies employ more representatives per head of prescribing population than universities employ teachers per pupil (www.nosuchthingasafreelunch.org). Although pharmaceutical companies claim to be research organisations they spend more on marketing and advertising than they do on research (NPC, 2002). Products are promoted by visits from representatives, gifts and other inducements such as funding for research, study days and lunches. It is important that nurse prescribers are aware that these inducements are all made with an ulterior motive and prescribers are reminded of the slogan that there is 'no such thing as a free lunch'. An American web page dedicated to these issues (www.nosuchthingasafreelunch.org) is a useful site to explore these issues and the evidence supporting them. The Associated Board of Pharmaceutical Industry Code of Practice (ABPI, 2001) regulates activities and advertising by pharmaceutical companies. Nurses, of course, are bound by their own code of conduct (NMC, 2002), which requires the nurse to be trustworthy and not to be seen to be promoting goods or services: nurses must not allow professional judgement to be influenced by commercial considerations.

## Medicines management

Medicines management aims to maximise health gain by making optimal use of medicines (NPC, 2002). In a sense, nurses have always been involved in medicines management so this concept is not new to them. The ability to prescribe puts the nurse more firmly in the driving seat of the medicines management initiative and increases her/his responsibility. Medicines management involves a range of interventions starting with prescribing, administration, and assessment of adverse effects and review of clinical and cost effectiveness. Many medicines management initiatives have been implemented across the country in order to deliver the *NHS Plan*'s targets (NHS, 2002), such as the national collaborative medicines management services programme hosted by the National Prescribing Centre and the community pharmacy medicines management project. These schemes aim to improve medicines management and nurse prescribers will inevitably become involved in the implementation process.

## Prescribing support in primary care trusts (PCTs)
David Spence

### Background

Structural changes in the NHS during the late 1980s and early 1990s resulted in the introduction of professional advisors (medical, pharmaceutical and nursing) at health authority level. Given that prescribing is the single most used intervention in health care in the UK, at a cost of £6.4 billion per year, it was not long before prescribing featured high on the priorities of the 'new' advisors.

In 1994, the audit commission published a report into prescribing in primary care (Audit Commission, 1994). This report criticises the lack of cost effectiveness, evidence and review within general practice prescribing. In 1995, the Department of Health set up a number of prescribing support pilots aimed at examining different models for support to general practice. Around this time, independent consultancies emerged who would provide considerable expertise to practices (mainly in the form of trained pharmacists), wishing to meet the challenges set out by the audit commission.

**The role of pharmacists**

As a profession, pharmacists find themselves ideally placed to conduct this type of work: their knowledge of drugs, clinical training and cost awareness coupled with their abilities to digest PACT (prescribing and cost data produced by the prescription pricing authority) saw them engaged by health authorities and individual practices alike.

By mid- to late-1997, a number of health authorities had appointed pharmacist prescribing advisors, utilising different models to support GP practices.

In 1998, the NHS Executive and National Prescribing Centre published *GP Prescribing Support,* a resource document and guide to the NHS (NPC, 1998). The release of this document coincided with the formation of primary care groups and copies were distributed widely within these organisations. This resulted in additional prescribing support being resourced within these organisations.

At health authority level, pharmaceutical advisors co-ordinated and managed the work of prescribing advisors and some distinctions started to emerge with respect to the type of work undertaken. *Table 7.1* lists the different roles which have emerged in recent years for pharmacists and technicians working in prescribing support.

**Prescribing support in context**

Early models for prescribing support included all the elements identified by the audit commission, ie. repeat prescribing and review. For many, however, it was the cost element which was stark and which brought about the success of pharmacists working in prescribing support.

Even now some primary care trusts are convinced that the main focus of prescribing support is to reduce and contain prescribing costs. Health economic models would question the sustainability of making cost efficiencies in the long term, in other words, they are not limitless. *Figure 7.1* illustrates this.

A good example to illustrate this would be generic prescribing; this is the proportion of prescription drugs prescribed by the proper chemical substance or generic name, as prices for these are mostly less than their brand name equivalent, there can be significant savings. The current national rate is 76%, having risen from around the mid 60% only a few years ago, the theoretical maximum for generic prescribing is between 70% and 80%. This is because it is considered high risk to prescribe some drugs using their generic name, for example, contraceptives; also, there are a number of drugs which should be consistently prescribed by brand in order to maintain appropriate levels in patients taking them, eg. epileptic drugs. Given that the national average for generic prescribing is nearing the theoretical maximum it is clear that there will only be in future a limited number of savings to be made from generic prescribing and the scope of the practice to improve upon its generic prescribing is reduced from what it was five years ago. Nevertheless, drugs continue to come off patent and it is important for PCTs that they are aware which drugs will be coming off patent so that they can ensure that they are prescribing generically from day one.

**Figure 7.1: Generic prescribing**

Prescribing support is more complex than simply reducing cost. Of more interest is the quality of prescribing and there exist a number of indicators of prescribing which are used in an attempt to capture how appropriate a practitioner's prescribing is, either relative to local peers or nationally. The appropriateness of prescribing becomes even more relevant when you consider the national service frameworks (NSF) and the work of the National Institute of Clinical Excellence (NICE) in improving the quality and accessibility of medicines. In addition, it is becoming clear that prescribing forms only one part of a developing and overarching medicines management agenda, which is focused on improving the patient's experience of medicine taking and various initiatives: for example, the national collaboratives are now underway to develop medicines management services (NPC, 2002).

| Table 7.1: Different roles of pharmacists and technicians in prescribing support |
| --- |

❖ **Pharmaceutical advisor**

Mostly experienced pharmacists with a good primary or secondary care background engaged in a range of strategic duties, resource management with responsibility for service delivery, including prescribing support.

❖ **Prescribing advisor**

These are pharmacists working to support practices in a specialised role utilising analytical, communication and technical expertise to achieve and improve prescribing practice and performance. Prescribing advisors conduct and co-ordinate work in a number of practices as well as the PCT function, eg. monitoring and implementation of PCT strategy.

❖ **Practice pharmacist**

This is a pharmacist working predominantly in a small number of practices. Work includes prescribing support, but may undertake additional duties on behalf of the practice such as medication review clinics.

❖ **Prescribing technician**

These posts are relatively new and growing in number. In the main, experienced pharmacy technicians have developed a range of roles to support practices in a similar way to prescribing advisors usually dealing with a more technical side of implementation of prescribing change.

❖ **Community pharmacist**

These are NHS independent contractors who provide dispensing services to the public, normally via separate premises. Like practice pharmacists, some community pharmacists have been engaged on a sessional basis supporting individual practices in a similar way to a practice pharmacist.

## Developing competencies

In April 2000, the roles of various pharmacists working in primary care were sufficiently diverse and the NHS Executive and National Prescribing Centre published a second document entitled, *Competencies for Pharmacists Working in Primary Care* (NPC, 2000). This document set out a number of levels of support, which could be undertaken within prescribing support role. Level 3 roles involved the strategic management of prescribing, normally envisaged to be at health authority level and essentially the pharmaceutical advisor role, including the management of prescribing incentive schemes, budget setting, service provision, monitoring data, developing strategic direction and formulary management, and the processes by which new drugs were introduced.

For Level 2 this was at the prescribing advisor level, involving facilitating change in prescribing at practice level, developing practice action plans and education material for the practice, reviewing repeat prescribing systems, conducting medication review and performing therapeutic switches.

Level 1, which arguably could now be fulfilled by prescribing technicians, was related to the day-to-day activity and processes involved in therapeutic switching, releasing prescribing advisors for increasing strategic roles.

The level of support available in PCTs is highly variable. When the competencies document was written it perceived some movement or changing role within primary care trusts. With some advisors having primary care trust only roles and some retaining health authority roles. In reality, the introduction of strategic health authorities has meant that most health authority pharmaceutical advisors were transferred to primary care trusts in a variety of guises, some retaining central supporting roles and some with primary care trust only roles.

## Summary

Prescribing support in primary care has developed rapidly and continues to diversify. Cost containment remains an important area and the growth in prescribing costs is of concern to primary care trusts, but work is underway in correcting more fundamental issues relating to medicines management. The role of pharmacists in providing prescribing support has been critical to success and the growth in numbers continues. However, more and more pharmacists will find themselves drawn into strategic management issues and the introduction of prescribing technicians and their developing supporting role is of significance, as will be the introduction of nurse prescribing advisors: individuals who could support the nurse prescribers extended and supplementary prescribing role.

## References

Adair J (1986) *Effective Teambuilding*. Gower Publishing, Aldershot

Association of the British Pharmaceutical Industry (2001) *Code of Practice for the British Pharmaceutical Industry*. Association of the British Pharmaceutical Industry, London

Audit Commission (1994) *A Prescription for Improvement. Toward more rational prescribing in general practice*. HMSO, London

Department of Health (2002) *Extending independent nurse prescribing within the NHS in England: A guide for implementation*. Crown Copyright. Department of Health publications, London

Klein J (1956) Building and maintaining high performance teams. In: Adair J, *Effective Teambuilding*. Gower Publishing, Aldershot: chap 9

NHS Executive and National Prescribing Centre (1998) *GP and Prescribing Support, a resource document and guide for the new NHS*. Online at: http://www.npc.co.uk (accessed 16 April 2003)

NHS Executive and National Prescribing Centre (2000) *Competencies for Pharmacists Working in Primary Care*. NPC, Liverpool

National Prescribing Centre (2001) Maintaining competency in prescribing: an outline framework to help nurse prescribers. 1st edn. NPC,

National Prescribing Centre (2002) *Medicines Management Collaborative programme*. Online at: http://www.npc.co.uk (accessed 16 April 2003)

Humphries J, Green J (2002) Nurse Prescribing. 2nd edn. Palgrave, London

Nursing and Midwifery Council (2002) *Standards for record keeping*. NMC, London

Shakespeare W (c 1600) *As you like it*. Act II, scene vii: 139–143

Skidmore (2002) Will you walk a little faster? In: Humphries J, Green J *Nurse Prescribing*. 2nd edn. Palgrave, London

# 8

# The future

One of the hardest fought battles of nursing (Jones, 1999) has been won, or has it? If we look back over the last twenty years, then the progress made in the development of nurse prescribing has, although slow at times, been remarkable. The current Government has pushed for nurses to take on the prescribing role, regarding it as a 'central plank' of the modernisation agenda (Hartley, 2003). Attitudes have shifted considerably despite some of the more negative attitudes voiced from minority sections of the medical domain, who consider nurse prescribing to be a dangerous and uncontrolled experiment (Horton, 2002). It is clear that a profession which is unresponsive to social change, will whither or be discarded, as it will lose the social approval on which it depends for its existence. Nurses have consistently retained the trust and approval of the British population, and the overprotective medical profession must learn to trust them too (While, 2002).

Fortunately for nursing, there are many medical colleagues who are supportive and realistic about the future development of patient care. New ways of working are becoming a reality and the old demarcations are being shattered (DoH, 2000). Some very committed doctors are providing excellent practice experiences for student nurse prescribers, and this activity is improving doctor/nurse relationships (Hartley, 2003). Indeed, the process of shifting tasks and roles between members of the different healthcare professions has, in many cases, been catalysed by acute staff shortages, reduced doctors' hours and clear evidence of nurses' ability to perform many of the roles previously carried out by doctors (Lissauer, 2003).

However, there are still challenges to face in overcoming some of the newer barriers to nurse prescribing. Firstly, the extended independent and supplementary prescribing course can be prohibitive in itself because of the demands it makes on the nurses who wish to train as prescribers. The logistics of releasing practice or specialist nurses, in particular, from the workplace is difficult. Potential nurse prescribers may be one of a small team of nurses, only employed on a part-time basis and releasing one nurse for twenty-six days to attend university, and providing twelve days supervision can mean that patient care is adversely affected. General practitioners who are busy already just cannot afford to release nurses for this length of time (Hartley, 2003). Nurse-led services in the acute sector sometimes have to run on a very depleted basis because specialist nurses cannot easily be replaced if nurses are away on courses.

The course also puts indirect pressure on the nurse colleagues who have to cover extra shifts in order to release the student prescriber to attend college. Specialist nurses are faced with similar pressures. They may be the only specialist nurse in the area. If they are not on duty they return from two days at college and a day with their supervisor, to find that they have to fit five days workload into two practice days. Local experience suggests that many students nurse prescribers, who spend their evenings catching up on visits, find that by the end of the course they are exhausted.

Some nurses from secondary care feel that the extended formulary is too limited to be of value to them, and find that supplementary prescribing does not really offer a viable alternative when patients are admitted during an acute phase of illness. The omission of controlled drugs from the supplementary prescribing remit, means that nurses involved in palliative care are still unable to give the autonomous care they need to give. In some cases, they still have to either put themselves into an unsafe position of accountability by taking a doctor's direction over the phone, or providing less than ideal care and comfort for the patient, while he or she waits for a doctor to sign a prescription for a stronger and much needed analgesic. Disease and discomfort unfortunately takes no account of staff shortages. The time taken for ministerial departments to make liberating decisions, which will allow nurses more autonomy to provide care for patients is, at times, tedious.

Changes to course delivery, using distance or online learning may improve accessibility for nurses as long as course content and quality of educational experience is not compromised. However, nurses may well find that they have to complete a larger proportion of the learning process in their own time. If this method of delivery is tried, these issues will need to be considered. Nurses will also need access to technology in line with their medical colleagues, who have convenient access to prescribing support systems and databases. Electronic patient records are easily accessible in the surgery, but to meet the needs of the nurse prescriber and provide the patient with the best care possible, they need to be accessible in all areas of the community. The provision, for example, of palm held or lap top computers which link to the GP practice is becoming more of an immediate need, but local experience suggests that practice is moving quicker than technology can keep pace with at the moment.

Nurses have always been a rare commodity: a fact that is even more evident at the present time. We have to raise the image of nursing to attract the calibre of recruits so desperately needed (Clegg, 2001). For many years, nursing has had the unfortunate image of, for example, the matronly Hatty Jaques of the 'Carry on' films, or the exhausted and confused nurses on soaps such as the popular 'Casualty' or 'ER' who have to forfeit their heroic job roles for disastrous private lives. Nurse prescribing is one way of raising, not only the image, but also the autonomy and job satisfaction of the nurse. Once in first level training the knowledge base needed by newly qualified nurses has to expand in relation to pharmacology, therapeutics and medicines management. Building blocks in pre-registration courses have to be firmly built. This will ensure that the nurses of tomorrow emerge from training as knowledgeable, potential future nurse prescribers (Mullally, 2003).

As non-medical prescribing, from disciplines such as pharmacy, dietetics and physiotherapy, becomes a reality, we should look forward to joint working. Multi-disciplinary education will help to facilitate better team working, with patients receiving prompt and appropriate treatment from whichever clinician is responsible for their care (Clegg, 2001). The future looks promising for patients: not only will greater access to medicines improve their quality of care, but more effective medicines management by the most appropriate prescribing practitioner involved will undoubtedly prove to be a safer and more effective use of resources.

Nurse prescribing is changing the landscape for patient care and the nursing profession will never be the same again (Cumberlege, 2003). Nurses now need to look at the way they deliver care to their patients and, if prescribing will enhance that care, they need to consider seriously joining the ever-increasing numbers of nurse prescribers.

## References

Clegg A (2001) Nurse prescribing empowers the new NHS. *Br J Community Nurs* **6**(1): 4

Cumberlege J (2003) A triumph of sense over tradition: the development of nurse prescribing. *Nurse Prescribing* **1**(1): 10–14

Department of Health (2000) *The NHS Plan, A plan for investment, A plan for reform*. The Stationery Office, London

Hartley J (2003) Nurse prescribing — the big picture. *Nurs Times* **99**(14): 23–7

Horton R (2002) *Nurse prescribing in the UK: right but also wrong*. Online at: http://wwwthelancet.com (accessed 19/9/02)

Jones M (1999) *Nurse Prescribing: Politics to Practice*. Ballière Tindall, London

Lissauer R (2003) Online at: http://www.ippr.org/research (accessed April 14th 2003)

Mullally S (2003) Keynote Presentation to the Association of Nurse Prescribers Annual Conference. Centennial Conference Centre, Birmingham

While A (2002) Nurses can be good substitutes. *Br J Community Nurs* **7**(7): 386

# Glossary of terms

| Term | Abbreviation | Description |
|------|--------------|-------------|
| Clinical supervision | | Clinical supervision is a practice-focused relationship involving an individual or a group of practitioners reflecting on practice, guided by a skilled supervisor |
| Controlled drugs | CDs | Preparations which are subject to the prescription requirements of the Misuse of Drugs regulations 1985. |
| Department of Health | DH | Government Department responsible for health care since 1997 |
| Department of Health | DHSS | Government Department and Social Security responsible for health and social care pre-1997 |
| District nurse | DN | A nurse who works in the community and who hold the qualification of specialist practitioner, district nurse |
| Health visitor | HV | A nurse who works in the community and who holds the qualification of specialist practitioner health visitor |
| Independent prescriber | | Doctor, dentist or vet |
| Independent nurse prescriber | NP | A nurse who has completed the district nurse or health visitor nurse prescribing course and is legally able to prescribe from the *Nurse Prescribers' Formulary* |
| Independent extended nurse prescriber | ENP | A nurse who has completed the independent extended nurse prescribing training course and who has an annotation to that effect on the Nursing and Midwifery Council Register |

| Term | Abbreviation | Description |
|------|-------------|-------------|
| Information technology | IT | Computer-generated information |
| Medications | | Medicines or drugs in either liquid, tablet or capsule form, injectable or taken orally |
| National Prescribing Centre | NPC | Prescribing support organisation |
| Over the counter | OTC | Any pharmaceutical item which may be bought over the counter without restriction |
| Patient group direction | PGD | A written direction relating to supply and administration of prescription only medicine by certain classes of healthcare professional |
| Pharmacy medicines | P Medicines | These items can only be sold over the counter under the supervision of a qualified pharmacist |
| Prescribe | | To order medications or other therapeutic items for a patient either using an FP10, a drug chart or similar or to verbally advise a patient to obtain the same |
| Prescription | FP10 | Form on which items are prescribed |
| Prescription only medicine | POM | Products which can only be obtained from a pharmacy by prescription |
| Prescription pricing authority | PPA | Organisation responsible for costing and reimbursing pharmacists for the costs of prescribable items |
| Royal College of Nursing | RCN | Professional organisation |
| Supplementary prescriber | SP | A nurse or pharmacist who has completed the independent extended and supplementary nurse prescribing training course and who has an annotation to that effect on the Nursing and Midwifery Council Register |

# Appendix I

Outline curriculum for the preparation of nurses, midwives and health visitors to prescribe from the Extended Nurse Prescribers' Formulary. This outline curriculum is separate from the preparation of district nurses and health visitors who prescribe from the *Nurse Prescribers' Formulary*.

## Entry requirements

All entrants to this education programme must meet the following requirements:

- valid registration on Part 1, 3, 5, 8, 10, 11, 12, 13, 14 or 15 of the Professional Register maintained by the United Kingdom Central Council for Nursing, Midwifery and Health Visiting;
- have appropriate experience in the area of practice in which they will be prescribing;
- an ability to study at academic level three;
- support from the employing organisation;
- have a designated medical practitioner who will provide the student with supervision, support and opportunities to develop competence in prescribing practice. (This includes shadowing opportunities.)

District nurses and health visitors who prescribe from the *Nurse Prescribers' Formulary*, and who, with local agreement, will extend their prescribing responsibilities under new arrangements from 2002, must complete this programme of preparation and meet the assessment requirements. It is expected that there will be recognition of prior learning and experience, where appropriate, to avoid duplication of learning.

## Aim

The education programme is to prepare nurses, midwives and health visitors to prescribe from the *Extended Nurse Prescribers' Formulary* as independent prescribers.

69

## Learning outcomes

The learning outcomes of the programme are at level three and will enable the practitioner to:

- undertake assessment and consultation with patients and carers;
- prescribe safely, appropriately and cost effectively;
- understand the legislation relevant to the practice of nurse prescribing;
- understand and use sources of information, advice and decision support in prescribing practice
- understand the influences on prescribing practice;
- apply knowledge of drug actions in prescribing practice;
- understand the roles and relationships of others involved in prescribing, supplying and administering medicines;
- practise within a framework of professional accountability and responsibility in relation to nurse prescribing.

## Indicative content

In order to meet the learning outcomes, it is expected that curriculum planning teams will include the following areas of study and develop these into a detailed curriculum which will enable practitioners to develop knowledge and competence as prescribers.

### Consultation, decision making and therapy, including referral

- ~ models of consultation
- ~ accurate assessment, communication and consultation with patients and their carers
- ~ concepts of working diagnosis or best formulation
- ~ development of a management plan
- ~ confirmation of diagnosis — further examination, investigation, referral for diagnosis
- ~ prescribe, not to prescribe, non-drug treatment or referral for treatment

### Influences on/and psychology of prescribing

- ~ patient demand versus patient need
- ~ external influences, for example, companies/colleagues
- ~ patient partnership in medicine-taking, including awareness of cultural and ethical needs

~ conformance — normalisation of professional prescribing behaviour
~ achieving shared understanding and negotiating a plan of action

**Prescribing in a team context**

~ national and local guidelines, protocols, policies, decision support systems and formulae — rationale, adherence to and deviation from
~ understand the role and function of other team members
~ documentation, with particular reference to communication between team members including electronic prescribing
~ auditing, monitoring and evaluating prescribing practice
~ interface between multiple prescribers and the management of potential conflict
~ budget/cost-effectiveness
~ issues relating to dispensing practices

**Clinical pharmacology including effects of co-morbidity**

~ pharmacology, including pharmacodynamics and pharmacokinetics
~ anatomy and physiology as applied to prescribing practice
~ basic principles of drugs to be prescribed – absorption, distribution, metabolism and excretion including adverse drug reactions (ADR), interactions and reactions
~ patient compliance and drug response
~ impact of physiological state in, for example, the elderly, young, pregnant or breast feeding women, on drug responses and safety

**Evidence-based practice and clinical governance in relation to nurse prescribing**

~ national and local guidelines, protocols, policies, decision support systems and formulae — rationale, adherence to and deviation from
~ continuing professional development — role of self and organisation
~ management of change
~ risk assessment and risk management, including safe storage, handling and disposal
~ clinical supervision
~ reflective practice
~ critical appraisal skills
~ auditing and systems monitoring
~ identifying and reporting ADRs and near misses

**Legal, policy and ethical aspects**

~ legal basis, liability and indemnity
~ legal implications of advice to self-medicate, including the use of complementary therapy and 'over the counter' (OTC) medicines
~ safe keeping of prescription pads, action if lost, writing prescriptions and record keeping
~ awareness and reporting of fraud
~ drug licensing
~ yellow card reporting to the Committee of Safety on Medicines (CSM)
~ prescribing in the policy context
~ manufacturers' guidance relating to literature, licensing and 'off-label'
~ ethical basis of intervention
~ informed consent, with particular reference to client groups in learning disability, mental health, children, the critically ill and emergency situations

**Professional accountability and responsibility**

~ UKCC *Code of Professional Conduct* and *Scope of Professional Practice*
~ accountability and responsibility for assessment, diagnosis and prescribing
~ maintaining professional knowledge and competence in relation to prescribing
~ accountability and responsibility to the employer

**Prescribing in the public health context**

~ duty to patients and society
~ policies regarding the use of antibiotics and vaccines
~ inappropriate use of medication including misuse, under- and over-use
~ inappropriate prescribing, over- and under-prescribing
~ access to healthcare provisions and medicines

## Teaching, learning and practice support strategies

It must be emphasised that self-directed learning and critical reflection are important component parts of the education process. The use of a portfolio or learning log as an effective means of facilitating and recording the student's critical thinking and reflection is well-established in professional education.

In addition, the use of random case analysis allows in-depth analysis of treatment scenarios where patient care and prescribing behaviour could be further examined and reflected upon. This approach also provides meaningful feedback to the student, the practice supporter and higher education.

The Board therefore expects these learning approaches to be used in the preparation of nurse prescribers.

The approved higher education institution must ensure that the designated medical practitioner who provides supervision, support and shadowing opportunities for the student is familiar with the requirements of the programme and, in particular, the achievement of the learning outcomes.

## Assessment strategies

Competence will be demonstrated through an assessment of theory and practice. To facilitate this, each student will maintain a portfolio of assessment and achievement of the stated learning outcomes.

The assessment requirements must be made explicit, in particular, the criteria for pass/fail and the details of the marking scheme.

A range of assessment strategies will be employed to test knowledge, decision-making and the application of theory to practice. These are:

a)   review of portfolio or learning log
b)   Objective Structured Clinical Examination (OSCE), a systematic and detailed examination of practice within a simulated learning environment such as a skills laboratory/centre
c)   satisfactory completion of the period of practice experience*
d)   written final examination consisting of:

(i)  multiple choice questions (MCQs)/short-answer questions — testing knowledge and application
(ii) essay — testing decision-making and prescribing behaviour

*The assessment of practice will be the responsibility of the prescribing medical practitioner providing support, teaching and supervision of the student.

## Length of the programme

The programme should be 25 days of contact time for the theory component, over a period of three months. In the period between these study days students are expected to shadow their prescribing medical practitioner for the equivalent of one day per week of educationally-led practice. The total length of the programme in both theory and practice is therefore approximately 37 days. It is anticipated that the programme will attract approximately 20 academic credits (CATS points) at level three.

# Appendix II

The Nursing and Midwifery Council's requirements for 'Extended independent nurse prescribing' and 'supplementary prescribing'

## Standard of programme

1    The standard of the programme should be no less than first degree level, such as to enable the registered nurse, midwife or health visitor, from parts 1, 3, 5, 8, 10, 11, 12, 13, 14, and 15, to acquire the competencies which are set out in section 8 of this paper.

2    A variety of assessment strategies should be employed to test knowledge and the application of theory to practice.

3    Assessment should focus upon the principles and practice of prescribing and professional accountability and responsibility of the practitioners on the Council's register undertaking the role.

## Kind of programme

4    The post-registration programme should be free-standing to meet the required competencies in practice.

5    Arrangements must be in place for teaching, supervision, support and assessment of the student prescriber in practice.

## Content of the programme

6    Pre-programme preparation:

    6.1    each individual registered nurse's, midwife's or health visitor's previous education, training and experience will influence the amount of pre-programme preparation required before embarking on the prescribing programme at academic level 3

    6.2    institutions may offer assessment of prior (experiential) learning (AP(E)L to accommodate those who are currently prescribing or, who may be able to demonstrate learning that is appropriate, to meet some of the competencies required of this standard

7    Content of the programme

    7.1    the content of the programme should reflect that prescribing is a competence-based professional activity. The underpinning knowledge requirements and competencies are outlined in Section 8 of this paper

    7.2    the content should reflect the requirements of local commissioners across the four countries of the United Kingdom in addition to those specified in this standard

8    The principal areas, knowledge and competencies required to underpin the practice of prescribing

| Principal areas | Knowledge | Competence |
|---|---|---|
| Principles | • Legislation that underpins prescribing | • Works within the legislative framework relevant to the area of practice and locality |
| | | • Understands the principles behind supplementary prescribing and how they are applied to practice |
| | • Team working principles and practice | • Awareness of the impact of prescribing in the wider delivery of care |
| | | • Able to work and communicate as part of a multidisciplinary prescribing workforce |
| | | • *Reviews diagnosis and generates treatment options within the clinical treatment management plan* |
| | • Philosophy and psychology of prescribing | • Understands the complexity of the external demands of influences on prescribing |
| Practice | • Up-to-date clinical and pharmaceutical knowledge | • Makes an accurate assessment and diagnosis and generates treatment options |
| | | • *Relevant to own area of expertise* |
| | • Principles of drug dosage, side-effects, reactions and interactions | • Able to prescribe safely, appropriately and cost effectively |
| | • Communication, consent and concordance | • *Understands how medicines are licensed, monitored* |
| | | • Able to work with patients and clients as partners in treatment |
| | | • Proactively develops dynamic clinical management plans |
| | | • Able to assess when to prescribe or make appropriate referral |
| | | • *Able to refer back to a medical practitioner when appropriate* |

|  |  |  |
|---|---|---|
|  | • Relationship of public health requirements to prescribing | • Aware of policies that have an impact on public health and influence prescribing practice<br>• Able to articulate the boundaries of prescribing practice in relation to the duty of care to patients and society |
| Accountability | • The *Code of Professional Conduct*<br><br>• The lines of accountability at all levels for prescribing<br><br><br>• Drug abuse and the potential for misuse<br><br>• Requirements of record keeping records<br>• Lines of communication | • Able to apply the principles of accountability to prescribing practice<br>• Able to account for the cost and effects of prescribing practice<br>• Regularly reviews evidence behind therapeutic strategies<br>• Able to assess risk to the public of inappropriate use of prescribed substances<br>• Understand where and how to access and use patient/client<br><br>• Able to write and maintain coherent records of prescribing practice<br>• Able to communicate effectively with patients, clients and professional colleagues |
| Responsibility | • Leadership skills<br><br>• Roles of other prescribers<br><br><br>• Relationship of prescribers to pharmacists<br><br>• Clinical governance requirements in prescribing practice<br><br><br>• Audit trails to inform prescribing practice | • Able to advise and guide peers in the practice of prescribing<br>• Able to articulate and understand the roles of other key stakeholders in prescribing practice<br>• Understand the requirements of pharmacists in the prescribing and supply process<br>• Link prescribing practice with evidence base, employer requirements and local formularies<br>• Demonstrate ability to audit practice, undertake reflective practice and identify continuing professional development needs |

# Index